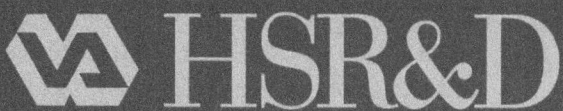

I0470839

Comparative Effectiveness of Smoking Cessation Treatments for Patients With Depression: A Systematic Review and Meta-analysis of the Evidence

November 2010

Prepared for:

Department of Veterans Affairs

Veterans Health Administration

Health Services Research & Development Service

Washington, DC 20420

Prepared by:

Evidence-based Synthesis Program (ESP) Center

Durham VA Medical Center

Durham, NC

John Williams, Jr., MD, MHSc, Director

Investigators:
Principal Investigator:
Jennifer M. Gierisch, PhD, MPH

Coinvestigators:
Lori A. Bastian, MD, MHSc
Patrick S. Calhoun, PhD
Jennifer R. McDuffie, PhD
John W. Williams, Jr., MD, MHSc

Medical Editor:
Liz Wing, MA

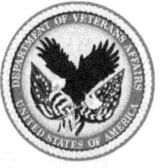

PREFACE

HSR&D's Evidence-based Synthesis Program (ESP) was established to provide timely and accurate syntheses of targeted healthcare topics of particular importance to VA managers and policymakers, as they work to improve the health and healthcare of Veterans. The ESP disseminates these reports throughout VA.

HSR&D provides funding for four ESP Centers and each Center has an active VA affiliation. The ESP Centers generate evidence syntheses on important clinical practice topics, and these reports help:

- develop clinical policies informed by evidence,

- the implementation of effective services to improve patient outcomes and to support VA clinical practice guidelines and performance measures, and

- set the direction for future research to address gaps in clinical knowledge.

In 2009, an ESP Coordinating Center was created to expand the capacity of HSR&D Central Office and the four ESP sites by developing and maintaining program processes. In addition, the Center established a Steering Committee comprised of HSR&D field-based investigators, VA Patient Care Services, Office of Quality and Performance, and VISN Clinical Management Officers. The Steering Committee provides program oversight and guides strategic planning, coordinates dissemination activities, and develops collaborations with VA leadership to identify new ESP topics of importance to Veterans and the VA healthcare system.

Comments on this evidence report are welcome and can be sent to Nicole Floyd, ESP Coordinating Center Program Manager, at nicole.floyd@va.gov.

Recommended citation: Gierisch JM, Bastian LA, Calhoun PS, McDuffie JR, Williams JW Jr. Comparative Effectiveness of Smoking Cessation Treatments for Patients With Depression: A Systematic Review and Meta-analysis of the Evidence. VA-ESP Project #09-010; 2010

This report is based on research conducted by the Evidence-based Synthesis Program (ESP) Center located at the Durham VA Medical Center, Durham, NC, funded by the Department of Veterans Affairs, Veterans Health Administration, Office of Research and Development, Health Services Research and Development. The findings and conclusions in this document are those of the author(s) who are responsible for its contents; the findings and conclusions do not necessarily represent the views of the Department of Veterans Affairs or the United States government. Therefore, no statement in this article should be construed as an official position of the Department of Veterans Affairs. No investigators have any affiliations or financial involvement (e.g., employment, consultancies, honoraria, stock ownership or options, expert testimony, grants or patents received or pending, or royalties) that conflict with material presented in the report.

TABLE OF CONTENTS

FIGURES

TABLES

EXECUTIVE SUMMARY

BACKGROUND

Smoking is disproportionately higher among persons with depression (45% versus 22%). Furthermore, smokers with depression may experience more challenges when trying to make and maintain a quit attempt, such as greater negative mood symptoms from withdrawal, higher nicotine dependence, and greater likelihood of relapse, than smokers without depression. Despite the complex relationship between tobacco use and depression, smokers with depression are motivated to quit smoking and should be offered cessation services. Several evidence-based smoking cessation treatments are effective for the general population of smokers. Yet the comparative effectiveness of these strategies in smokers with depression is uncertain. Also, it is uncertain if factors that may facilitate targeted interventions, such as depression status, gender, and treatment sequencing (i.e., concurrent versus sequential) for mood and smoking cessation, differentially impact the effectiveness of smoking cessation interventions. We conducted a systematic review of the peer-reviewed literature to answer the following key questions:

Key Question 1: For patients with a history of a depressive disorder or current significant depressive symptoms, what is the comparative effectiveness of different smoking cessation strategies on smoking abstinence rates?

Key Question 2: For patients with a history of a depressive disorder or current significant depressive symptoms, are there differential effects of smoking cessation strategies by depression status (i.e., history of MDD, current depressive symptoms, current MDD)?

Key Question 3: For patients with a history of a depressive disorder or current significant depressive symptoms, are there differential effects of smoking cessation strategies by gender?

Key Question 4: For patients with a history of a depressive disorder or current significant depressive symptoms, does treatment effectiveness differ by whether smoking cessation/ depression treatments are delivered concurrently or sequentially?

Key Question 5: What is the nature and frequency of adverse effects of smoking cessation treatments in patients with a history of a depressive disorder or current significant depressive symptoms?

This review was commissioned by the Department of Veterans Affairs' Evidence-based Synthesis Program. The topic was selected after a formal topic nomination and prioritization process that included representatives from the Office of Mental Health Services, Health Services Research and Development, the Mental Health QUERI, and the Office of Mental Health and Primary Care Integration. The key research questions for this review were developed and refined after preliminary review of published peer-reviewed literature and consultation with VA and non-VA experts to select the patients and subgroups, interventions, outcomes, and settings addressed in this review.

METHODS

We searched for English-language publications in MEDLINE® (via PubMed®), Embase®, PsycINFO®, and the Cochrane Library from database inception through March 10, 2010. We developed search strategies in consultation with a master librarian. Titles, abstracts, and articles were reviewed in duplicate by trained researchers. A trained researcher abstracted data from published reports into evidence tables; a second reviewer overread the evidence tables. When study designs and outcomes reported were similar, we estimated pooled risk ratios (RR) with 95% confidence intervals (CI) by using a random effects model with the Mantel-Haenszel method. For these analyses, we classified each intervention element into the following categories: antidepressants, nicotine replacement therapy (NRT), brief smoking cessation counseling, behavioral counseling for smoking cessation, or behavioral mood management treatment. All other data were narratively summarized.

RESULTS

We screened 884 titles, rejected 792, and performed full-text reviews on 92 articles. We manually pulled 6 additional papers in order to retrieve supplemental methodological or background information on studies included in the full-text review. Of these 98 papers, we excluded 75. The 23 included reports encompassed 16 unique trials, of which only three recruited participants with current depression.

Key Question 1: For patients with a history of a depressive disorder or current significant depressive symptoms, what is the comparative effectiveness of different smoking cessation strategies on smoking abstinence rates?

We identified three types of intervention strategies: cotreatments augmented with behavioral mood management treatment (six trials), cotreatments augmented with antidepressant therapy (five trials), and cotreatments augmented with NRT (four trials). Cotreatments generally consisted of some type of smoking cessation counseling (e.g., brief, behavioral), with or without NRT. We also identified three additional trials that used exercise behavioral counseling plus NRT, mailed self-help materials, or long-acting opiate antagonist plus behavioral counseling as smoking cessation interventions.

Pooled results from our meta-analysis demonstrate a small, positive effect of adding behavioral mood management treatments to smoking cessation cotreatments (RR = 1.45, 95% CI 1.01 to 2.07). All of the included antidepressant trials showed small, positive effects when comparing antidepressants plus behavioral counseling to placebo plus behavioral counseling, but a summary estimate of effect from meta-analysis was not statistically significant (RR = 1.31, 95% CI 0.73 to 2.34). We were unable to conduct a meta-analysis of NRT trials. Three of the four NRT trials showed positive effects with clinically significant abstinence. Two of these NRT trials reported statistically significant differences. Results from three of the four included studies suggest that offering NRT appears to have a small, positive effect on smoking cessation rates among smokers who are depressed. We found insufficient evidence to support exercise behavioral counseling, mailed self-help materials, or naltrexone, although both naltrexone and mailed self-help materials showed positive effects in single trials.

Key Question 2: For patients with a history of a depressive disorder or current significant depressive symptoms, are there differential effects of smoking cessation strategies by depression status (i.e., history of MDD, current depressive symptoms, current MDD)?

Only two studies provided information on differential effectiveness of smoking cessation intervention strategies by depression status. Study researchers conducted subgroup analysis only; no treatment by depression interaction effects were directly tested. Among participants who were history positive for unipolar depression in Evins (2008), 39% in the bupropion plus behavioral counseling plus NRT arm and 32% in the placebo plus behavioral counseling plus NRT control arm were abstinent at the end of trial (p-value NS). Bupropion did not significantly improve smoking cessation rates compared to active control condition for participants with current depression (33% versus 31%; p-value NS). In Munoz and colleagues (1997), the addition of mailed mood management content improved cessation rates over a mailed smoking cessation guide (38.5% versus 7.4%; p = 0.01) at 6 months postrandomization for participants with a history of major depressive episode (MDE). Smokers with current MDE did not experience significant differences (17.9% versus 8.0%; p = 0.15).

Key Question 3: For patients with a history of a depressive disorder or current significant depressive symptoms, are there differential effects of smoking cessation strategies by gender?

Only one included study reported a significant treatment by gender interaction among study participants with a history of or current depression. Covey and colleagues (1999) found a significant treatment by gender by depression interaction. Women with past histories of MDD experienced higher quit rates when randomized to receive naltrexone in combination with six sessions of individual behavioral counseling compared to women with depression receiving placebo control at 6 months. Men who were MDD history positive did not have higher quit rates on naltrexone.

Key Question 4: For patients with a history of a depressive disorder or current significant depressive symptoms, does treatment effectiveness differ by whether smoking cessation/ depression treatments are delivered concurrently or sequentially?

No studies directly compared smoking cessation and depression treatments delivered concurrently versus sequentially.

Key Question 5: What is the nature and frequency of adverse effects of smoking cessation treatments in patients with a history of a depressive disorder or current significant depressive symptoms?

Most included trials did not provide information on the nature and frequency of adverse effects of treatments. Of the five studies that reported adverse effects, three provided some level of detail about the magnitude and significance of adverse effects. These three studies all evaluated the addition of antidepressants with other smoking cessation treatments. In two of the three studies, selected adverse effects were more common in patients randomized to antidepressants compared to placebo control.

FUTURE RESEARCH RECOMMENDATIONS

While this review provided some evidence of smoking cessation strategies for patients with depression, more work is needed in this area. Principally, we found very little trial data on intervening with smokers with current depression. Future studies should be designed to test smoking cessation interventions for this vulnerable population. Next, within the trials we identified, we found little research on key moderators that may influence treatment effectiveness (e.g., gender, depression status). Moderator analysis will facilitate subgroup identification and may lead to better treatment matching. In many instances, we were able to address only the incremental benefit of adding one strategy to an intervention package (e.g., behavioral counseling with or without antidepressant). Future studies should be designed to allow for direct comparisons between combinations of likely efficacious therapies for smokers with depression such as combination NRT therapy. Also, we were unable to disaggregate multicomponent interventions. Future research should be designed to disentangle active ingredients of interventions and optimize dose, duration, frequency, and sequencing of smoking cessation strategies. Finally, future research should be conducted to characterize adverse effects of treatments, including changes in negative affect and depressive symptoms.

CONCLUSIONS

In conclusion, the peer-reviewed literature contained few randomized controlled trials of smoking cessation interventions for patients with depression. Most trials excluded patients with current or recent MDD. Thus, most of the data for this evidence review were from subgroup analyses of patients with depressive symptoms or remote histories of depressive disorder. However, the majority of reports included in this evidence review were of good quality and had consistent results. We found insufficient evidence to characterize adverse effects of treatments and examine moderator effects of gender, depression status, and treatment delivery sequencing.

However, this evidence review lends support for several promising interventions. Our results support a small, positive effect for adding behavioral mood management counseling to smoking cessation cotreatments. Smokers with depression may respond better to smoking cessation interventions augmented with mood management techniques. Evidence also shows support for adding NRT; however, included trials were too varied to be analyzed quantitatively. All of the included antidepressant trials showed small, positive effects, but a summary estimate of effect was not statistically significant. However, there was heterogeneity in antidepressant type across studies. Effects likely vary with medication type. Health care providers should consider encouraging their patients with depression who smoke to seek smoking cessation services that include NRT and also address behavioral mood management counseling.

EVIDENCE REPORT

INTRODUCTION

Tobacco smoking is the single greatest preventable cause of disease in the United States.[1,2] Half of all American smokers who fail to quit will die of a smoking-related illness.[3] Cigarette use is higher among Americans with depression than in the general U.S. population.[4] Persons with depression are about twice as likely (45% versus 22%) to be current smokers than are individuals who are not depressed,[5] and smokers are more likely to have a history of depression.[6,7] Moreover, veterans have higher rates of depression and smoking compared to the general population.[8-12]

Several hypotheses have been offered to explicate the association between smoking and depression, including mood-enhancing effects of nicotine[13,14] and common genetic and environmental factors. Depression also appears to be an important factor in smoking cessation.[15-20] Smokers who are depressed are more likely to relapse from a quit attempt, have higher nicotine dependence, suffer negative mood symptoms from withdrawal, and suffer greater smoking-related morbidity and mortality than the general population of smokers.[17,18,21-24]

Smokers with depression are highly motivated to quit smoking.[7,25] One study found that 79% of smokers with depression intended to quit, with 24% ready to make a quit attempt in the next month.[26] Despite the complex relationship between tobacco use and depression, smokers with depression should be offered cessation services.[27,28] Several evidence-based smoking cessation intervention strategies exist for the general population of smokers.[29-35] All forms of nicotine replacement therapy (NRT) (e.g., gum, transdermal patch, inhaler, lozenges) augment successful quit attempts, increasing quit rates by as much as 50 to 70%.[35] Also, use of some antidepressants (i.e., bupropion, nortriptyline) can double the chances of smoking cessation, and this effect seems independent of the antidepressive effects of these medications.[36] For behavioral interventions, there is a strong dose-response relationship between treatment intensity and smoking cessation rates.[37] More intensive interventions, measured by total contact time, are associated with increased abstinence rates. For example, smoking cessation counseling improves quit attempts over self-help aids and other less intensive therapies.[29,33,34,38] Combining behavioral interventions with pharmacotherapy increases quit attempts over each therapy delivered alone and is considered the gold standard of care for effective smoking cessation treatment.[29,37,39]

Gender, depression status (e.g., history positive, depression symptom severity), and content delivery timing (i.e., sequential, concurrent) may differentially impact the effectiveness of smoking cessation intervention efforts for smokers with depression. When trying to quit smoking, women who are depressed may experience more difficulty with withdrawal symptoms and, consequently, higher rates of smoking relapse to alleviate withdrawal symptoms compared to their male smoker counterparts.[40] Level of depressive symptoms or depression type may influence patients' ability to make and maintain quit attempts.[17,18,22] Also, smokers with depression may benefit from smoking cessation programs that target both depression symptoms and tobacco use. However, it is not known if these two conditions should be treated concurrently or sequentially. For example, it is not known if treating depression first influences smoking cessation treatment effectiveness. Treating depression first may lead to greater treatment adherence and, consequently, better cessation rates. It is plausible but unstudied. Smokers with psychiatric comorbidities may benefit from combined behavioral counseling and pharmacotherapy with longer therapeutic smoking cessation approaches (i.e., exceeding 8 to 12 weeks) to reduce likelihood of dropout and depression relapse.[27,41] However, no systematic reviews have synthesized the comparative effectiveness of smoking cessation strategies for persons with depressive symptoms. Many unanswered questions remain about how effective smoking cessation interventions are for adults with depression.

METHODS

TOPIC DEVELOPMENT

This review was commissioned by the Department of Veterans Affairs' Evidence-based Synthesis Program. The topic was selected after a formal topic nomination and prioritization process that included representatives from the Office of Mental Health Services, Health Services Research and Development, the Mental Health QUERI, and the Office of Mental Health and Primary Care Integration. The key research questions for this review were developed and refined after preliminary review of published peer-reviewed literature and consultation with VA and non-VA experts to select the patients and subgroups, interventions, outcomes, and settings addressed in this review.

The final key questions were as follows:

Key Question 1: For patients with a history of a depressive disorder or current significant depressive symptoms, what is the comparative effectiveness of different smoking cessation strategies on smoking abstinence rates?

Key Question 2: For patients with a history of a depressive disorder or current significant depressive symptoms, are there differential effects of smoking cessation strategies by depression status (i.e., history of MDD, current depressive symptoms, current MDD)?

Key Question 3: For patients with a history of a depressive disorder or current significant depressive symptoms, are there differential effects of smoking cessation strategies by gender?

Key Question 4: For patients with a history of a depressive disorder or current significant depressive symptoms, does treatment effectiveness differ by whether smoking cessation/ depression treatments are delivered concurrently or sequentially?

Key Question 5: What is the nature and frequency of adverse effects of smoking cessation treatments in patients with a history of a depressive disorder or current significant depressive symptoms?

We developed and followed a standard protocol for all steps of this review. Our approach was guided by the analytic framework shown in Figure 1.

Figure 1. Analytic Framework

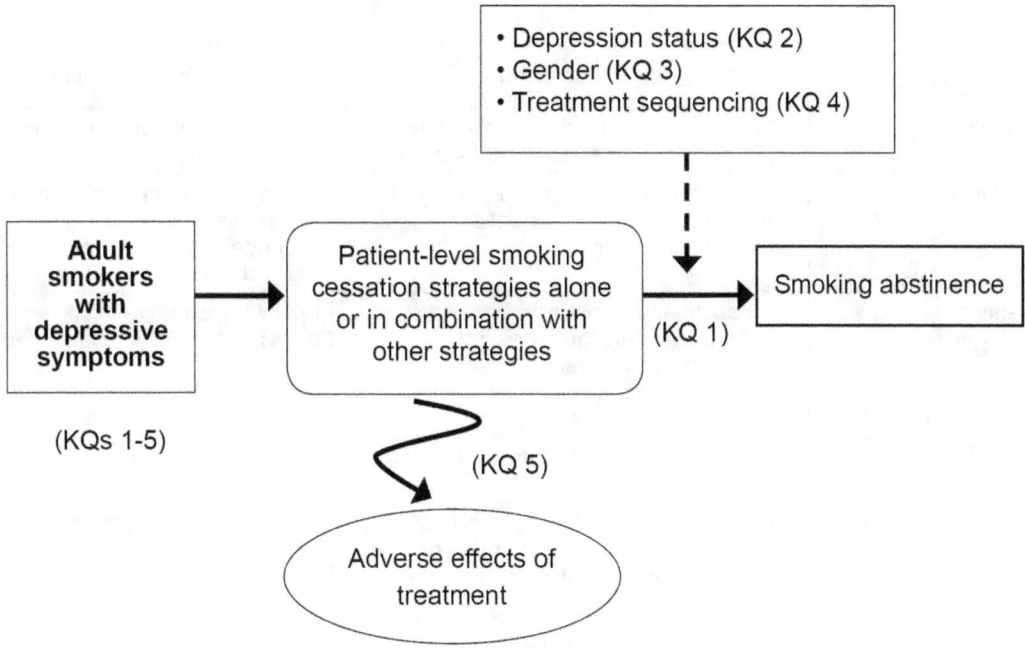

SEARCH STRATEGY

We searched for English-language publications in MEDLINE (via PubMed), Embase, PsycINFO, and the Cochrane Library from database inception through March 10, 2010. We developed search strategies in consultation with a master librarian. The search terms and MeSH headings for the search strategies appear in Appendix A. We supplemented electronic searching by examining the bibliographies of included studies.

STUDY SELECTION

Using prespecified inclusion/exclusion criteria, two trained researchers reviewed the list of titles and selected articles for further review. Each article retrieved was reviewed with a brief screening form used to determine eligibility. To be included in our evidence report, a study had to (1) be a randomized controlled trial (RCT), (2) compare two or more smoking cessation interventions or compare intervention to control, and (3) report smoking cessation outcomes in adults with depression. Detailed eligibility criteria are described in Table 1.

Table 1. Summary of Inclusion and Exclusion Criteria

Study characteristic	Inclusion criteria	Exclusion criteria
Study design	RCTs or a secondary data analysis from RCTs of smoking cessation interventions	Non-English language publication, cross-sectional studies
Population	Adults age 18 and over with a history of a depressive disorder or current significant depressive symptoms[a]	Pregnant women, adolescents, postpartum depression, depressive symptoms secondary to another primary condition (e.g., substance abuse, schizophrenia)
Interventions	Any patient-level smoking cessation strategies (e.g., self-help, quit lines, physician or brief advice, behavioral counseling, pharmacologic therapies) alone or in combination with other strategies	Policy-level interventions (e.g., smoking bans), mass media campaigns
Comparators	Active comparators or control (e.g., usual care or placebo)	None
Setting	Outpatient (e.g., mental health clinics, primary care) or delivered through remote communication technologies (e.g., telephone, Web)	Hospital-based (inpatient) interventions
Outcome	KQs 1-4: Smoking abstinence reported at ≥ 3 months postrandomization KQ 5: Adverse effects including behavioral symptoms, increased anxiety, depression[b]	Relapse prevention[c]

[a] We define significant depressive symptoms as meeting a designated threshold on a validated assessment instrument (e.g., CES-D, BDI).

[b] We considered depression as an adverse effect when participants moved from depressive symptoms to a depressive disorder, or when the intervention arm showed significantly more depressive symptoms compared to a decrease in symptoms in the comparator condition.

[c] Intervention strategies that reduce the likelihood of recent quitters returning to smoking.

Abbreviations: BDI = Beck Depression Inventory, CES-D = Center for Epidemiologic Studies-Depression Scale, RCT = randomized controlled trial

DATA ABSTRACTION

A trained researcher abstracted data from published reports into evidence tables; a second reviewer overread the evidence tables. We resolved disagreements by consensus among the first and second reviewer or by obtaining a third reviewer's opinion when consensus could not be reached. We abstracted the following data from included studies: (1) Study design and setting, (2) eligibility criteria, (3) exclusion criteria, (4) sample size, (5) demographics, (6) duration of follow-up, (7) depression clinical category, (8) baseline smoking characteristics (e.g., cigarettes per day, tobacco dependence), (9) method used to assess depression, (10) intervention characteristics (e.g., mode, frequency, dose, core therapy components), (11) outcome measures, (12) results, and (13) adverse effects.

QUALITY ASSESSMENT

We assessed risk of bias using the key quality criteria described in the Agency for Healthcare Research and Quality (AHRQ) *Methods Guide for Effectiveness and Comparative Effectiveness Reviews* (hereafter referred to as the *General Methods Guide*),[42] adapted for this specific topic. We abstracted data on adequacy of randomization and allocation concealment, comparability of groups at baseline, blinding, completeness of follow-up and differential loss to follow-up, whether incomplete data were addressed appropriately, validity of outcome measures, and conflict of interest. Using these data elements, we assigned a summary quality score of Good, Fair, or Poor to individual RCTs.

DATA SYNTHESIS

We constructed evidence tables showing the study characteristics and results for all included studies, organized by key question and intervention, as appropriate. We critically analyzed studies to compare their characteristics, methods, and findings. We compiled a summary of findings for each key question.

When study designs and outcomes reported were similar, we estimated pooled risk ratios with 95% confidence intervals (CIs) by using a random effects model with the Mantel-Haenszel method. For these analyses, we classified each intervention element into the following categories: Antidepressants, nicotine replacement therapy (NRT), brief smoking cessation counseling, behavioral counseling for smoking cessation, or behavioral mood management treatment. We defined brief smoking cessation counseling as counseling that was similar in content to what may be given during a physician visit. We defined behavioral counseling for smoking cessation as multisession individual or group therapy that used behavioral strategies, such as those common in cognitive behavioral therapy (CBT), to influence tobacco use. Behavioral mood management treatment was defined as group or individual counseling intended to influence negative mood and improve depression symptomatology above and beyond standard smoking cessation counseling.

Using these intervention categories, there were sufficient studies to perform meta-analyses for two comparisons: Mood management versus control and antidepressants versus control. Other comparisons were synthesized qualitatively. All studies that were analyzed quantitatively used behavioral counseling for smoking cessation in the intervention and control arms. For the mood management comparison, we subgrouped studies using NRT alone or in combination with antidepressants.

The primary outcome was smoking abstinence without smoking relapse. Smoking abstinence was defined as smoking cessation collected as (1) point prevalence abstinence (e.g., in past 7 days) or (2) extended abstinence (e.g., since quit date or last previous follow-up). We included only one effect size per study. Therefore, we assessed the most distal and rigorous (extended abstinence over point prevalence) outcomes reported and categorized as short-term ($3 < 6$ months) or long-term (≥ 6 months) confirmed by self-report, biochemical validation, or both. Our outcome was informed by outcomes used in the Cochrane Collaborative reviews, which are based on the Russell Standard.[43] The U.S. Department of Health and Human Services Tobacco Use and Dependence Guideline Panel recommended a minimum of a 6-month period to assess treatment differences in the longer term.[37] Therefore, we used 6 months or longer outcomes for meta-analyses. Abstinence could be assessed by self-report or with biochemical verification.

Two studies[44,45] used a factorial design to compare pharmacological and behavioral interventions; these comparisons were treated as separate studies in the analyses. We evaluated heterogeneity visually and with the Cochran Q statistic[46] using a threshold p-value of less than 0.10[47] and the I^2 statistic.[48] We considered I^2 statistic thresholds of 0% to 40%, 30% to 60%, 50% to 90%, and 75% to 100% to represent between-study heterogeneity that might not be important, moderate, substantial, or considerable, respectively.[49] We planned a priori to conduct subgroup analyses by depression status (severity and specific diagnosis), gender, and treatment sequencing, but there were not sufficient studies to conduct these analyses. All analyses were performed using Review Manager 5.0 software (The Cochrane Collaboration, Oxford).

Grading the Evidence for Each Key Question

We graded the strength of evidence for each key question using the principles from the GRADE Working Group.[50] In brief, this approach assesses the strength of evidence for each critical outcome by considering risk of bias, consistency, directness, precision, and publication bias. Other domains relevant to observational designs were not pertinent to our review. After considering each domain, a summary rating of High, Moderate, Low, or Insufficient strength of evidence was assigned after discussion by two reviewers (Table 2).

Table 2. Definitions for Strength of Evidence Rating

Strength of evidence rating	Definition
High quality	Further research is very unlikely to change our confidence in the estimate of effect
Moderate quality	Further research is likely to have an important impact on our confidence in the estimate of effect and may change the estimate
Low quality	Further research is very likely to have an important impact on our confidence in the estimate of effect and is likely to change the estimate
Insufficient	Evidence on an outcome is absent or too weak, sparse or inconsistent to estimate an effect

PEER REVIEW

Peer reviewer comments and our responses are presented in Appendix B.

RESULTS

LITERATURE SEARCH AND STUDY CHARACTERISTICS

The combined literature search of PubMed, Embase, PsycINFO, and Cochrane databases, minus duplicates, contained 884 unique citations, of which we excluded 792 after reviewing titles and abstracts. We then conducted full-text reviews of 92 articles and pulled 6 additional papers in order to retrieve supplemental methodological or background information on studies included in the full-text review. Of these 98 papers, we excluded 75. Figure 2 summarizes the literature flow. The 23 included reports encompassed 16 unique trials with a total of 3,553 depressed and nondepressed participants. Table 3 summarizes study characteristics. In studies that included depressed and nondepressed participants, we report information for the depressed subgroup when available.

Figure 2. Literature Flow Diagram

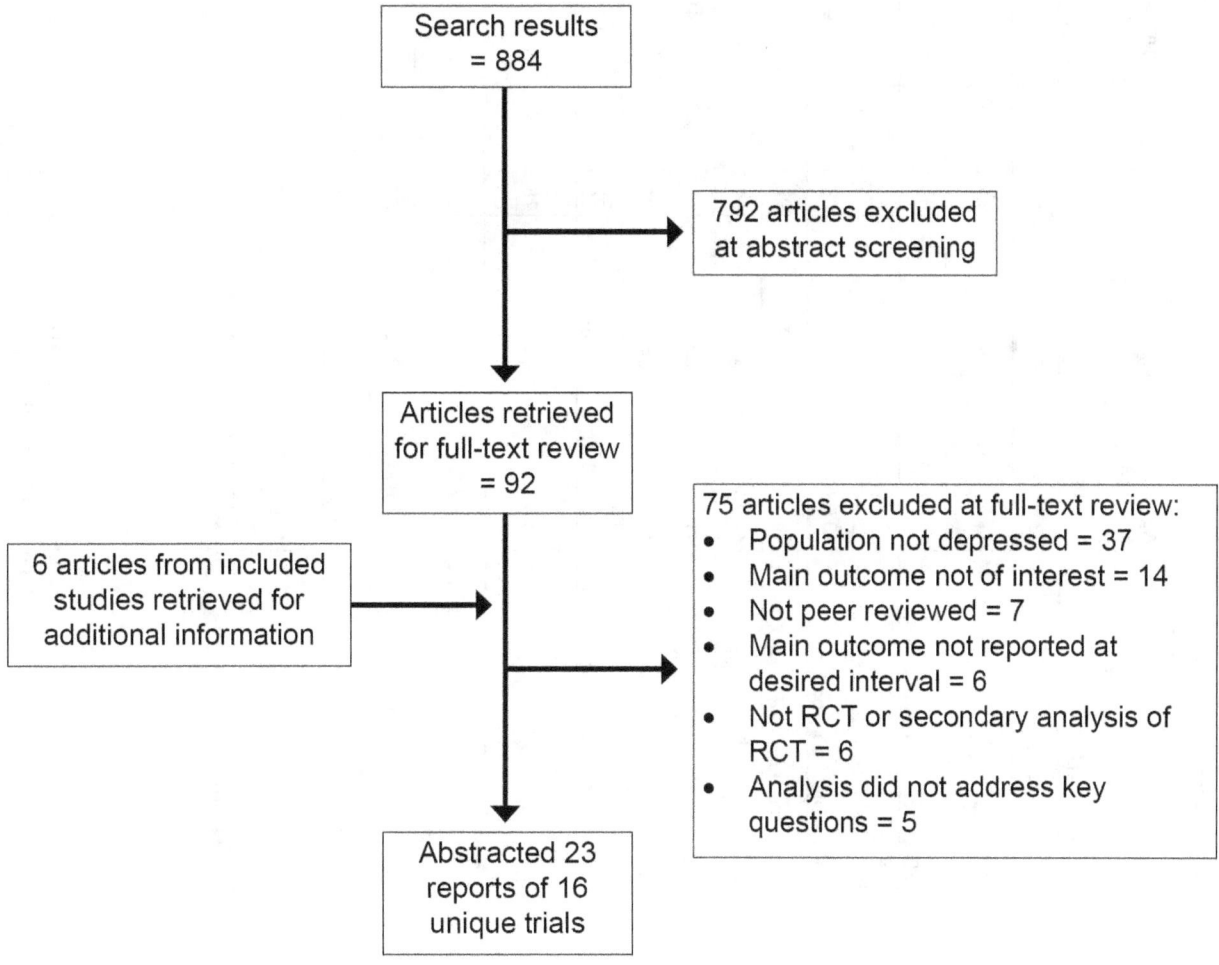

Comparative Effectiveness of Smoking Cessation Treatments for Patients With Depression

Table 3. Summary of Study Characteristics

Study, year	Study quality[a]	Sample size	Age Mean (SD)	% Female	% White	FTND Mean (SD)	Cigarettes per day Mean (SD)	Depressed mood at baseline Mean (SD)
Brown, 2001	Good	179 All MDD history positive	45.1 (9.3)	59.8	97.2	6.8 (1.9)	NR	BDI: 7.8 (6.31)
Covey, 1999	Fair	80 45% MDD history positive	33.8[b] (8.2)	68.0[b]	NR	NR	30.3 (10.1)	NR
Covey, 2002	Good	134 All MDD history positive	44.5 (10.7)	63.4	87.3	6.1(2.4)[b]	NR	BDI: 8.0 (7.7) CES-D: 14.9 (10.8) HDRS: 4.8 (4.4)
Duffy, 2006	Good	184 35% depressed smokers	57.0 (9.9)	16.0	90.0	NR	NR	NR
Evins, 2008	Good	199 All MDD history positive	43.0 (11.0)	49.0	NR	5.8 (2.2)	25.0 (11)	HDRS: 10.6 (6.3)
Hall, 1994	Fair	149 31% MDD history positive	40.6 (9.2)	52.0	88.0	6.4 (1.9)	24.9 (10.9)	BDI: 6.4 (5.9)[c]
Hall, 1996	Fair	201 22% MDD history positive	39.7 (NR)	52.0	92.0	NR	23.8 (9.8)	BDI: 6.7 (5.4)
Hall, 1998	Good	199 33% MDD history positive	41.9[c] (9.9)	42.0[c]	59.0[c]	5.5 (2.2)[c]	21.8 (10.4)[c]	BDI: 12.1 (8.3)[c]
Hall, 2006	Good	322 All with current depression	41.5[b] (12.4)	69.6	68.3	3.8 (2.4)	15.8 (10.0)	BDI: 20.6 (11.7)[b]
Hayford, 1999	Good	615 19% MDD history positive	42.2 – 43.7[d]	54.6	96	FTQ: 7.1-7.3 (1.7)[d]	26.2(8.5) – 27.5(9.6)[d]	BDI: 4.1(4.2) –4.7 (5.0)[d]
Kinnunen, 1996	Good	269 34% met criteria for depression	40.4 (12.6) 41.6[c] (12.7)	51.0 61.0[c]	82.0 80.0[c]	5.6 (2.4)[c]	22 (10.4)[c]	NR
Kinnunen, 2008	Good	608 32% met criteria for depression	38.5 (11.3)[c]	51.0[c]	78.6[c]	Women: 5.6(2.3)[c] Men: 6.2 (2.3)[c]	Women: 21.0(10.0)[c] men:26.6(11.7)[c]	CES-D: Women: 24.8(7.0)[c] Men: 24.4 (6.9)[c]
MacPherson, 2010	Good	68 All with mildly elevated depressive symptoms	45.0 (12.2)[b]	48.5 (NR)	27.3	5.8 (1.8)[b]	18.8 (7.1)[b]	BDI: 10.8 (5.2)[b]
Munoz, 1997	Fair	136 78% MDE history positive	35.3 (NR)	38.2	0.0	NR	14.1 (8.2)	CES-D: 21.3 (13.9)
Saules, 2004	Fair	150 20% MDD history positive	39.8 (NR)	54.5	73.2	5.9 (NR)	NR	BDI: 4.92 (NR)
Vickers, 2009	Fair	60 All with current depression	41.8 (12.1)[b]	100.0	98.0[b]	NR	21.6 (11.1)[b]	HRSD: 12.8 (6.0) CES-D: 29.8 (9.3)

[a] Study quality assessed via key quality criteria described in AHRQ's General Methods Guide.

[b] Mean for intervention arm only.

[c] Mean for depressed subgroup.

[d] Range of means from randomized groups at baseline.

Abbreviations: BDI = Beck Depression Inventory, CES-D = Center for Epidemiologic Studies-Depression Scale, FTQ = Fagerstrom Tolerance Questionnaire, FTND = Fagerstrom Test for Nicotine Dependence, HDRS = Hamilton Depression Rating Scale, NR = not reported, MDD = major depressive disorder; MDE = major depressive episode

Most studies were of good quality according to quality criteria described in AHRQ's *General Methods Guide*.[42] All studies were conducted in the U.S. with English-speaking participants except one, which was conducted with Spanish speakers living in the U.S.[51] All reports, except one,[52] reported smoking cessation outcomes for at least 6 months from the start of the trial. Most studies excluded participants with current MDD; however, 19 to 78% of participants in these studies had a history of MDD or exceeded a screening threshold for significant depressive symptoms. Of the studies that recruited smokers with depression, three recruited MDD history-positive participants,[53-55] two recruited participants with current depression as measured by the CES-D[56] or the PRIME-MD,[57] and one recruited participants with mildly elevated depressive symptoms as assessed by the BDI-II.[58] For the remainder of this report, we refer to depression as (1) significant depressive symptoms as measured by validated assessment instrument (e.g., CES-D, BDI) or (2) a history of MDD.

KEY QUESTION 1. For patients with a history of a depressive disorder or current significant depressive symptoms, what is the comparative effectiveness of different smoking cessation strategies on smoking abstinence rates?

Intervention Types

All but two interventions tested combination therapies consisting of some type of counseling and pharmacotherapy.[51,53] Of the studies that included behavioral counseling, the most common therapy was CBT conducted in person via small group or individual therapy. Only one included study conducted behavioral counseling via telephone.[59] Six studies included a behavioral mood management treatment.[44,45,53,58-60] Mood management treatments ranged from smoking cessation–focused behavioral counseling augmented with one-time additional mood management counseling to intensive multisession group or individual CBT counseling. One study included mood management content delivered via mailed print materials.[51] Of the studies that included antidepressant pharmacotherapies, four used bupropion,[55,57,59,61] and three tested some other antidepressant (i.e., sertraline, fluoxetine, nortriptyline).[45,54,62] Of studies that included antidepressants, two used NRT as a cotreatment,[55,62] and two used NRT as a first-line therapy before offering bupropion.[57,59] One study tested behavioral counseling plus a pill formulation of a long-acting opiate antagonist, naltrexone, as a smoking cessation aid.[63] No studies using varenicline were identified that met our eligibility criteria. Below, we summarize the evidence for smoking cessation interventions for adults with depression. When able, we conducted meta-analysis to quantitatively summarize evidence of comparative effectiveness of interventions.

Comparative Effectiveness of Smoking Cessation Strategies

NRT + Brief counseling versus placebo + brief counseling. Two studies of good quality compared the addition of nicotine gum to brief counseling compared to brief counseling plus placebo (Table 4).[52,64] Kinnunen and colleagues (1996) compared the addition of 2 or 4 mg of nicotine gum to one-time brief counseling. Participants were advised to use the gum ad lib, with a target range of 9 to 15 pieces a day. In a subgroup analysis of participants with significant depressive symptoms as measured via the CES-D (n = 93), smokers with depression receiving either active gum dose were more likely to quit smoking than smokers with depression receiving placebo gum (29.5% versus 12.5%; p-value NR) at 3 months post–quit date. In another trial, Kinnunen and colleagues (2008) reported the long-term effects of adding 2 or 4 mg of nicotine gum to 9 sessions of brief, 5- to 10-minute counseling sessions. Among participants with depression (n = 196), smokers receiving nicotine gum were more likely to remain abstinent at 12 month post–quit date than were smokers receiving placebo gum (15.1% versus 5.7%; p = 0.01).

Table 4. Smoking Cessation Studies of NRT Plus Brief Counseling Versus Placebo Plus Brief Counseling

Study, year	Intervention	Comparator	Follow-up duration
Kinnunen, 1996	Nicotine gum + one-time brief individual behavioral counseling	Placebo gum + one-time brief individual behavioral counseling	3 months
Kinnunen, 2008	Nicotine gum + 9 brief in-person individual counseling sessions	Placebo gum + 9 brief in-person individual counseling sessions	12 months

NRT + Behavioral counseling versus active control. Two studies compared the addition of NRT to behavioral counseling.[44,57] In a two-by-two factorial design, Hall and colleagues (1996) compared nicotine gum to placebo gum with 10 sessions of group CBT smoking cessation counseling versus 10 sessions of health education (Table 5). Analyses were collapsed across treatment arms. Participants were given 2 mg nicotine gum or placebo gum starting at counseling session three and instructed to chew one piece per hour, 12 hours per day for the next 8 weeks. At Week 8, participants were given enough gum to taper treatment over the next 4 weeks. Smoking status was obtained and confirmed with biological assessments at Weeks 8, 12, 26, and 52. For MDD history-positive participants (n = 88), 22% receiving nicotine gum were abstinent compared to 33% receiving placebo gum at 52 weeks (p-value NR). This study was of fair quality due to omission of several key quality indicators (i.e., follow-up rates, randomization and allocation procedures, baseline characteristics).

In a study of good quality, Hall and colleagues (2006) offered nicotine patches plus 6 weeks of individual staged-care CBT behavioral counseling and computerized motivational feedback (Table 5). All participants had a current diagnosis of depression based on the PRIME-MD. Counseling sessions lasted 30 minutes and took place over 8 weeks. Participants were offered 21 mg patches for the first 6 weeks, 14 mg patches for the following 2 weeks, and then offered 7 mg patches for an additional 2 weeks. If patients did not quit smoking with NRT or relapsed during treatment, patients could request bupropion. A brief contact and smoking cessation referral served as the control condition. Smoking status was confirmed at 3, 6, 12, and 18 months postrandomization by expired carbon monoxide at ≤ 10 ppm. Staged-care counseling condition plus NRT outperformed brief contact control over time (OR = 4.55, 95% CI 1.04 to 19.93) with abstinence rates of 14.11% and 9.43% at 12 months and 18.4% and 13.21% at 18 months for the intervention and control, respectively.

Table 5. Smoking Cessation Studies of NRT Plus Behavioral Counseling Versus Active Control

Study, year	Intervention	Comparator	Follow-up duration
Hall, 1996[a]	Nicotine gum + 10 sessions of group CBT smoking cessation counseling or 10 session health education	Placebo gum 10 sessions of group CBT smoking cessation counseling or 10 sessions health education	12 month
Hall, 2006	Transdermal nicotine patch (or bupropion if failed NRT) + staged motivational feedback + 6 sessions of individual CBT smoking cessation counseling	Brief contact + list of referrals to smoking cessation programs and stop smoking guide	18 months

[a] Factorial design and analysis collapsed across treatment arms.

Synthesis of Evidence on NRT

Four studies addressed comparative effectiveness of adding single-form NRT (i.e., not combination NRT therapy) to other cotreatments versus an active control for adults with depression. Most trials reported smoking cessation outcomes of 12 months or greater from point of randomization. Of the four studies included in this review, only one intervened with adults with current depression;[57] results of other studies are from subgroup analyses. Cotreatments were heterogeneous and ranged from intensive CBT counseling to brief one-time counseling. However, most studies were of good quality and reported a small, positive effect for the use of NRT.

Antidepressant therapy + cotreatment versus placebo + cotreatment. Five trials reported results of adding antidepressants to cotreatments compared to active control condition for smokers with depression. Three of these studies, all of good quality and involving 255 smokers with depression, provided 6-month or greater outcomes data and were included in a meta-analysis.[45,54,61] These studies compared antidepressants plus behavioral counseling to behavioral counseling plus placebo (Table 6). Two studies compared antidepressant therapy plus a cotreatment of behavioral counseling and NRT. These studies reported outcomes less than 6 months postrandomization and were not included in the meta-analysis.

Table 6. Smoking Cessation Studies of Antidepressant Therapy Plus Behavioral Counseling Versus Placebo Plus Behavioral Counseling

Study, year	Intervention	Comparator	Follow-up duration
Covey, 2002	Sertraline + 9 individual in-person smoking cessation behavioral counseling sessions augmented with supportive approach to manage negative affect associated with quitting smoking	Placebo + 9 individual in-person smoking cessation behavioral counseling sessions augmented with supportive approach to manage negative affect associated with quitting smoking	34 weeks
Hall, 1998[a]	Nortriptyline + 10 session of group CBT smoking cessation counseling or 10 session health education	Placebo + 10 session of group CBT smoking cessation counseling or 10 session health education	64 weeks
Hayford, 1999	Bupropion + 11 brief in-person individual counseling sessions	Placebo + 11 brief in-person individual counseling sessions	12 months

[a] Factorial design and analysis collapsed across treatment arms.

Participants receiving antidepressants plus behavioral counseling were not more likely to be abstinent compared to participants receiving behavioral counseling plus placebo at 6-month postrandomization (RR = 1.31, 95% CI 0.73 to 2.34, Cochran Q = 0.55, p = 0.76, I^2 = 0%) (Figure 3).

Figure 3. Risk of Smoking Cessation at Least 6 Months After Start of Antidepressant Therapy Plus Behavioral Counseling Compared With Placebo + Behavioral Counseling

Study or Subgroup	Antidepressant Events	Total	Placebo Events	Total	Weight	Risk Ratio M-H, Random, 95% CI
Hayford 1999	4	28	2	28	13.0%	2.00 [0.40, 10.05]
Hall 1998b	7	32	7	33	39.4%	1.03 [0.41, 2.61]
Covey 2002	11	66	8	68	47.5%	1.42 [0.61, 3.30]
Total (95% CI)		126		129	100.0%	1.31 [0.73, 2.34]
Total events	22		17			

Heterogeneity: Tau² = 0.00; Chi² = 0.55, df = 2 (P = 0.76); I² = 0%
Test for overall effect: Z = 0.90 (P = 0.37)

In a study of good quality, Evins and colleagues (2008) tested the efficacy of adding 12 weeks of bupropion to a cotreatment consisting of 8 weeks of transdermal NRT and 13 sessions of group CBT smoking cessation counseling (Table 7).[55] All participants had a lifetime history of unipolar depressive disorder (UDD). Results were in the expected direction, favoring antidepressant use in combination with behavioral counseling plus NRT over behavioral counseling plus NRT alone (36% versus 31%; p-value NR). However, participants randomized to receive bupropion were no more likely to achieve smoking abstinence at end of treatment in intention-to-treat (ITT) analysis with dropouts considered smokers. Moreover, smoking abstinence was associated with depressive symptoms, regardless of antidepressant use.

Saules and colleagues (2004) also tested the addition of an antidepressant to a cotreatment of NRT and behavioral counseling (Table 7).[62] This study was of fair quality. Participants in the intervention arm received 10 weeks of transdermal NRT plus 14 weeks of either 20 or 40 mg of fluoxetine in combination with 6 weeks of group CBT smoking cessation counseling. Again, results were in the expected direction and favored the addition of antidepressant therapy. However, among participants who were history positive for MDD (n = 30), Saules found no significant differences in abstinence rates when fluoxetine was added to NRT and intensive behavioral counseling.

Table 7. Smoking Cessation Studies of Antidepressant Therapy Plus Behavioral Counseling Plus NRT Versus Placebo Plus Behavioral Counseling Plus NRT

Study, year	Intervention	Comparator	Follow-up duration
Evins, 2008	Bupropion + 13 group CBT smoking cessation counseling + NRT patch	Placebo + 13 group CBT smoking cessation counseling + NRT patch	13 weeks
Saules, 2004	Fluoxetine + 6 group CBT smoking cessation counseling + NRT patch	Placebo + 6 group CBT smoking cessation counseling + NRT patch	12 months

Synthesis of Evidence on Antidepressants

Five studies addressed comparative effectiveness of adding antidepressants to other cotreatments versus an active control (e.g., counseling + NRT + placebo) for adults with depression. For included studies, antidepressants were prescribed at therapeutic doses. Only two included studies recruited participants with histories of MDD;[54,55] results of other studies are from subgroup analyses. All cotreatments included multisession counseling, and four studies were of good quality. However, there was heterogeneity in antidepressant type across included studies. Only one used bupropion, the only antidepressant with an FDA indication for smoking cessation. Overall, we did not find enough evidence to support adding antidepressants to other smoking cessation cotreatments in order to improve smoking cessation rates among persons with depression.

Mood management treatment + cotreatment versus cotreatment/active control. Six trials reported results of adding mood management treatments to behavioral counseling (Table 8). Other cotreatments given to all participants include NRT,[44,58-60] nortriptyline,[45] or NRT plus bupropion or paroxetine.[59] Five of these studies, involving 402 smokers with depression, provided sufficient data for meta-analysis.[44,45,53,58,60]

Table 8. Smoking Cessation Studies With a Mood Management Treatment Component

Study, year	Intervention	Comparator	Follow-up duration
Mood management treatment + behavioral counseling versus behavioral counseling			
Brown, 2001	8 group sessions of depression and smoking cessation CBT	8 group sessions of smoking cessation CBT	12 months
Mood management treatment + behavioral counseling + NRT versus behavioral counseling + NRT			
Hall, 1994	5 group sessions of CBT mood management + 5 group sessions of smoking cessation counseling + nicotine gum	5 group sessions of smoking cessation counseling + nicotine gum	52 weeks
Hall, 1996[a]	5 group sessions of CBT mood management + 5 group sessions of smoking cessation counseling + nicotine gum	10 sessions of standard group smoking cessation health education + nicotine gum	52 weeks
MacPherson, 2010	8 group sessions of smoking cessation CBT that included behavioral activation therapy + NRT patch	8 group sessions of smoking cessation CBT + NRT patch	26 weeks
Mood management treatment + behavioral counseling + NRT/antidepressant versus control			
Duffy, 2006	9 to 11 sessions of combined smoking, depression, alcohol abuse telephone CBT + bupropion + NRT (if failed bupropion monotherapy in the past) OR NRT + paroxetine (if failed bupropion in the past for depression)	One-time behavioral counseling and referral to appropriate services for substance use/abuse and/or depression	6 months
Hall, 1998[a]	5 group sessions of CBT mood management + 5 group sessions of smoking cessation counseling + nortriptyline or placebo	10 session health education + nortriptyline or placebo	64 weeks

[a] Factorial design and analysis collapsed across treatment arms.

All studies included in the meta-analysis were in the expected direction, favoring the addition of mood management treatment to smoking cessation cotreatments (RR = 1.45, 95% CI 1.01 to 2.07, Cochran Q = 2.16, p = 0.71, I^2 = 0%). Subgroup analysis suggests smoking cessation may be more likely when mood management treatment was added to cotreatments that included NRT or antidepressants in addition to behavioral counseling (RR = 1.66, 95% CI 0.95 to 2.90, Cochran Q = 1.8, p = 0.62, I^2 = 0%) (Figure 4). However, confidence intervals overlap, and this contrast was not statistically significant.

Figure 4. Risk of Smoking Cessation at Least 6 Months After Start of Mood Management Treatment Plus Cotreatment Compared to Active Control

Study or Subgroup	Mood Management		Control		Weight	Risk Ratio M-H, Random, 95% CI	Risk Ratio M-H, Random, 95% CI
	Events	Total	Events	Total			
NRT or Antidepressant							
MacPherson 2010	5	35	0	33	1.6%	10.39 [0.60, 180.84]	
Hall 1994	10	29	4	17	13.0%	1.47 [0.54, 3.96]	
Hall 1996a	7	21	5	23	13.3%	1.53 [0.57, 4.10]	
Hall 1998a	9	34	5	31	13.4%	1.64 [0.62, 4.37]	
Subtotal (95% CI)		119		104	41.2%	1.66 [0.95, 2.90]	
Total events	31		14				

Heterogeneity: Tau² = 0.00; Chi² = 1.80, df = 3 (P = 0.62); I² = 0%
Test for overall effect: Z = 1.79 (P = 0.07)

No NRT or Antidepressant							
Brown 2001	28	86	23	93	58.8%	1.32 [0.83, 2.10]	
Subtotal (95% CI)		86		93	58.8%	1.32 [0.83, 2.10]	
Total events	28		23				

Heterogeneity: Not applicable
Test for overall effect: Z = 1.15 (P = 0.25)

Total (95% CI)		205		197	100.0%	1.45 [1.01, 2.07]	
Total events	59		37				

Heterogeneity: Tau² = 0.00; Chi² = 2.16, df = 4 (P = 0.71); I² = 0%
Test for overall effect: Z = 2.03 (P = 0.04)

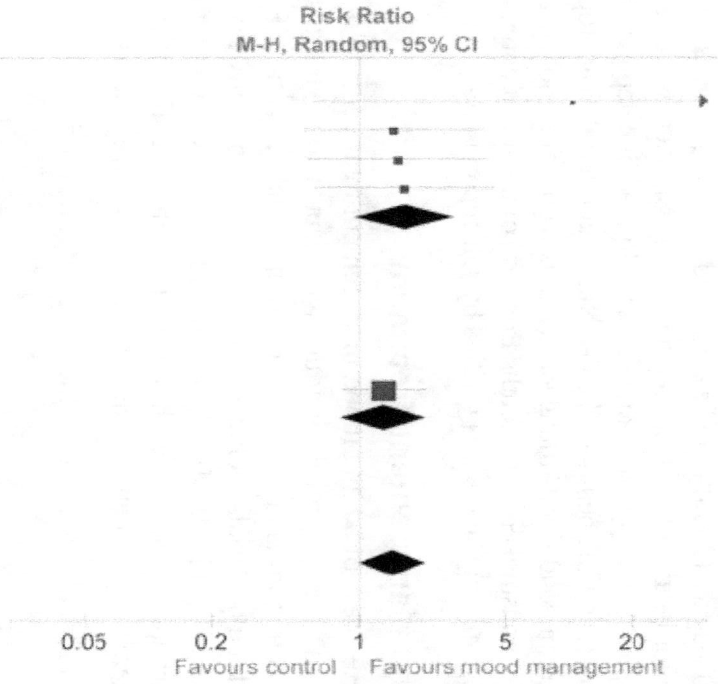

19

In a study of good quality, Duffy and colleagues (2006) tested a combined smoking, depression, and alcohol abuse CBT counseling protocol for head-and-neck cancer survivors.[59] Smokers who were depressed were offered NRT and bupropion or paroxetine. Content was delivered by telephone over the course of 9 to 11 counseling sessions. One-time behavioral counseling and referral to appropriate follow-up services served as the comparator condition. Among participants who were smokers and depressed at baseline (n = 64), 51% were nonsmokers at 6 months from end of treatment compared to 17% in the control arm (p-value NR). Smoking status was verified by self-report only.

Synthesis of Evidence on Mood Management Treatment

Six trials addressed comparative effectiveness of adding mood management treatments to other smoking cessation cotreatments versus an active control for adults with depression. All trials reported smoking cessation outcomes at 6 months or greater from point of randomization. Four of these trials were of good quality. Of the five trials included in the meta-analysis, only two studies recruited participants with either a history of MDD[53] or elevated depressive symptoms.[58] Results of other studies are from subgroup analyses. Overall, results indicate a small, positive effect for the addition of mood management treatment to smoking cessation cotreatments.

Other intervention strategies. Three additional trials tested other types of interventions. These are summarized below and in Table 9.

In a study of fair quality, Covey and colleagues (1999) tested behavioral counseling plus a long-acting opiate antagonist, naltrexone, as a smoking cessation aid.[63] Participants received six individual brief behavioral counseling sessions. Participants in the control arm received the same counseling plus placebo. Smoking status was verified by blood cotinine level of < 15 ng/ml. Of the 36 participants with a history of MDD, results favored use of naltrexone in combination with counseling over counseling plus placebo (28.6% versus 9.1%; p-value NR).

Munoz and colleagues (1997) tested the efficacy of a self-administered mood management intervention plus smoking cessation guide compared to a smoking cessation guide alone delivered through the mail for Spanish-speaking smokers.[51] To be eligible for the trial, participants needed to indicate that they were either "completely" or "very" sure they wanted to quit smoking in the next 3 months. The smoking cessation guide was a 36-page booklet from the National Cancer Institute and contained tips on how to quit smoking. The mood management treatment consisted of relaxation exercises, self-monitoring booklet, and pleasant activity guide. An audio cassette explained how to use the materials. Among participants with a history of MDE, the addition of mailed mood management content improved cessation rates over the mailed smoking cessation guide (38.5% versus 7.4%; p = 0.01) at 6 months postrandomization. For smokers with current MDE, no significant differences were found (17.9% versus 8.0%; p = 0.15). This study was of fair quality.

In another fair study, Vickers and colleagues (2009) conducted a small randomized pilot to test the feasibility of behavioral counseling to promote exercise as a smoking cessation intervention for depressed female smokers.[56] Women were randomized to receive brief smoking cessation counseling plus 6 weeks of transdermal NRT, plus either 10 weeks of CBT to encourage exercise or a health education contact control condition. The intervention was feasible but did not significantly improve smoking cessation rates compared to the health education control (17% versus 23%; p = 0.75).

Table 9. Other Smoking Cessation Intervention Strategies Studies

Study, year	Intervention	Comparison	Follow-up duration
Covey, 1999	Naltrexone + 6 individual in-person behavioral counseling sessions	Placebo + 6 individual in-person behavioral counseling sessions	6 months
Munoz, 1997	Mailed smoking cessation guide + mood management guide	Mailed smoking cessation guide + mood management guide at 3 months delayed	6 months
Vickers, 2009	10 in-person individual exercise counseling sessions that include brief smoking cessation counseling + NRT	10 in-person individual health education sessions that include brief smoking cessation counseling + NRT	24 weeks

Synthesis of Evidence on Other Intervention Strategies

We identified three other types of smoking cessation strategies, each with only one RCT. Covey and colleagues (1999) and Munoz both reported positive results for participants with depression. However, studies were of fair quality (e.g., no ITT analysis, lack of detail on study measures, randomization and allocation concealment procedures not well described) and with select populations (e.g., Spanish speakers), which limits confidence in the estimates of effects and applicability of results to other populations. Results of Vickers and colleagues (2009) demonstrated no effect for using exercise counseling as a smoking cessation intervention strategy for smokers with depression.

KEY QUESTION 2. For patients with a history of a depressive disorder or current significant depressive symptoms, are there differential effects of smoking cessation strategies by depression status (i.e., history of MDD, current depressive symptoms, current MDD)?

Only two studies provided sufficient information to report differential effectiveness of smoking cessation intervention strategies by depression status. For both reports, study researchers conducted subgroup analysis only; no treatment by depression interaction effects were directly tested.

Evins and colleagues (2008) recruited 199 smokers who had a lifetime diagnosis of UDD. Participants were randomized to 12 weeks of bupropion versus placebo. Both groups received a cotreatment consisting of 8 weeks of transdermal NRT and 13 sessions of group CBT smoking cessation counseling.[55] Among participants who were history positive for unipolar depression (n = 109), 39% in the bupropion arm and 32% in the control arm were abstinent at the end of trial (p-value NS). Among participants with current depression (n = 90), bupropion did not significantly improve smoking cessation rates compared to cotreatment control condition (33% versus 31%; p-value NS).

Munoz and colleagues (1997) tested the efficacy of a mailed self-administered mood management intervention plus smoking cessation guide compared to only a smoking cessation guide for Spanish-speaking smokers.[51] The addition of mailed mood management content improved cessation rates over the mailed smoking cessation guide (38.5% versus 7.4%; p = 0.01) at 6 months postrandomization for participants with a history of MDE. Smokers with current MDE did not experience significant differences (17.9% versus 8.0%; p = 0.15).

KEY QUESTION 3. For patients with a history of a depressive disorder or current significant depressive symptoms, are there differential effects of smoking cessation strategies by gender?

Only one included study reported a significant treatment by gender interaction among study participants with a history of or current depression.[63] Covey and colleagues (1999) found a significant treatment by gender by depression interaction. Women with past histories of MDD (n = 26) experienced higher quit rates when randomized to receive naltrexone in combination with six sessions of individual behavioral counseling compared to women with depression receiving placebo control at 6 months (22.2% versus 0%; p = 0.04). Men with past histories of MDD (n = 10) did not experience significantly higher quit rates with naltrexone at 6 months.

KEY QUESTION 4: For patients with a history of a depressive disorder or current significant depressive symptoms, does treatment effectiveness differ by whether smoking cessation/depression treatments are delivered concurrently or sequentially?

No studies directly compared smoking cessation and depression treatments delivered concurrently versus sequentially.

KEY QUESTION 5: What is the nature and frequency of adverse effects of smoking cessation treatments in patients with a history of a depressive disorder or current significant depressive symptoms?

Table 10 details reported adverse effects of the 16 included trials. Overall, 11 studies did not provide information on the nature and frequency of adverse effects of treatments. Of the five studies that reported adverse effects, three provided some level of detail about the magnitude and significance of adverse effects; other studies reported too few cases to conduct statistical tests. These three studies all evaluated the addition of antidepressants with other smoking cessation treatments. In two of the three studies, selected adverse effects were more common in patients randomized to antidepressants.

Table 10 also summarizes change in depressive symptoms from baseline to follow-up when comparing intervention and control arms among participants classified as depressed at baseline. Seven trials did not report changes in depressive symptoms from baseline to follow-up per arm for participants classified as depressed at study entry. Six studies reported no significant differences. Of three studies that reported significant differences, only Vickers and colleagues (2009) reported more favorable changes in depressive symptoms associated with the control arm compared to the intervention arm. Kinnunen and colleagues (1996) and MacPherson and colleagues (2010) reported more favorable changes in depressive symptoms associated with the intervention arms.

Table 10. Adverse Effects of Included Studies

Study, year	Intervention	Adverse effects reported[a] (% reported in intervention versus control)	Change in depressive symptoms[b]
Brown, 2001	8 group sessions of depression and smoking cessation CBT	NR	No difference between intervention and control arms
Covey, 1999	Naltrexone + 6 individual in-person behavioral counseling sessions	Panic attack, malaise, sleepless-ness, concentration difficulty, nausea and vomiting, disoriented and shaky, spaciness, dizzy, abdominal pain, lightheadedness, shortness of breath	NR
Covey, 2002	Sertraline + 9 individual in-person smoking cessation behavioral counseling sessions augmented with supportive approach to manage negative affect associated with quitting smoking	NR	No difference between intervention and control arms
Duffy, 2006	9 to 11 sessions of combined smoking, depression, alcohol abuse telephone CBT + bupropion + NRT (if failed bupropion monotherapy in the past) OR NRT + paroxetine (if failed bupropion in the past for depression)	NR	No difference between intervention and control arms
Evins, 2008	Bupropion + 13 group sessions of CBT smoking cessation counseling + NRT patch	NR	No difference between intervention and control arms
Hall, 1994	5 group sessions of CBT mood management + 5 group sessions of smoking cessation counseling + nicotine gum	NR	NR
Hall, 1996	5 group sessions of CBT mood management + 5 group sessions of smoking cessation counseling + nicotine gum	NR	No difference between intervention and control arms
Hall, 1998	5 group sessions of CBT mood management + 5 group sessions of smoking cessation counseling + nortriptyline	Dry mouth (78% vs 33%)[c], lightheadedness (49% vs 22%)[c], shaky hands (23% vs 11%)[c], blurry vision (16% vs 6%)[c]	NR
Hall, 2006	Transdermal nicotine patch (or bupropion if failed NRT) + staged motivational feedback + 6 sessions of individual CBT smoking cessation counseling	NR	No difference between intervention and control arms
Hayford, 1999	Bupropion + 11 brief in-person individual counseling sessions	Headache (29% vs 31-33%), insomnia (21% vs 30-35%)[c], rhinitis (17% vs 10 to 12%), dry mouth (5% vs 13%)[c], increased anxiety (11% vs 5-7%)	NR
Kinnunen, 1996	Nicotine gum + one-time brief individual behavioral counseling	NR	Decrease in NRT gum arm and no change in placebo arm

Study, year	Intervention	Adverse effects reported[a] (% reported in intervention versus control)	Change in depressive symptoms[b]
Kinnunen, 2008	Nicotine gum + 9 brief in-person individual counseling sessions	Heart palpitations, nausea, vomiting, dizziness, breathing difficulties, tongue blisters, damage to dental work, sore jaw[d]	NR
MacPherson, 2010	8 group sessions of smoking cessation CBT that included behavioral activation therapy + NRT patch	NR	Greater decrease in intervention arm compared to control arm
Munoz, 1997	Mailed smoking cessation guide + mood management guide	NR	NR
Saules, 2004	Fluoxetine + 6 group sessions of CBT smoking cessation counseling + NRT patch	Adverse effects not more common in intervention arms but did not list types	NR
Vickers, 2009	10 in-person individual exercise counseling sessions that include brief smoking cessation counseling + NRT	NR	Decrease in health education arm and increase in exercise counseling arm

[a] Adverse effects reported for all subjects in trial.

[b] For participants within depressed subgroup, statistically significant change in depressive symptoms from baseline to follow-up.

[c] Statistically significant and greater proportion affected in intervention arm compared to proportion affected in control arm.

[d] Less than 2% of low-nicotine dependent and 6% of high-nicotine dependent participants in the intervention arms experienced most common NRT gum adverse effects (i.e., heart palpitations, nausea, vomiting, dizziness).

Abbreviations: CBT = cognitive behavioral therapy, NR = not reported, NRT = nicotine replacement therapy

DISCUSSION

SUMMARY AND DISCUSSION

There is a synergistic and potentially bidirectional relationship between depression and smoking.[6,14,19,65,66] Smokers with depression are significantly less likely to quit smoking, and depressed individuals are more likely to be smokers.[5-7] Consequently, there is a need to identify effective smoking cessation interventions for this disproportionately affected population. We conducted a systematic review of smoking cessation intervention strategies for persons with depression. We also sought to examine differential effects of smoking cessation treatment by depression status, gender, and treatment sequencing and to characterize adverse effects of smoking cessation treatments in patients with depression. We found insufficient evidence to examine moderator effects and to characterize adverse effects. However, findings suggest several promising smoking cessation strategies for persons with depression. We summarize and discuss our findings here.

We identified three types of intervention strategies: cotreatments augmented with behavioral mood management treatment (six trials), cotreatments augmented with antidepressant therapy (five trials), and cotreatments augmented with NRT (four trials). Cotreatments generally consisted of some type of smoking cessation counseling (e.g., brief, behavioral), with or without NRT. We also identified three additional trials that used behavioral counseling to promote exercise plus NRT,[67] mailed self-help materials,[51] or long-acting opiate antagonists plus behavioral counseling[63] as smoking cessation interventions. Overall, we found insufficient evidence to support exercise behavioral counseling, mailed self-help materials, or naltrexone as smoking cessation strategies for smokers with depression. Although both naltrexone and mailed self-help materials showed positive effects in single trials, further study is required to assess the efficacy of these strategies. Also, it is possible that we may have missed studies with unpublished but relevant data.

We did not identify any studies using varenicline that met our eligibility criteria. Varenicline stimulates dopamine release, which reduces nicotine cravings and withdrawal symptoms, and blocks nicotine receptors, which may reduce the pleasurable effects of continued nicotine usage. Pooled results of two RCTs showed significantly higher abstinence rates at the end of 12 weeks of varenicline treatment compared to both placebo and bupropion.[68,69] However, given the latest concerns about mental health instability within the veteran population,[70] varenicline should be reserved for special cases and will require close observation.

Smokers with depression are more likely to have increased levels of negative mood both precessation and postcessation.[15,71-73] Also, negative mood is associated with greater relapse rates.[74,75] Mood management therapy may serve to moderate negative mood associated with making and maintaining a quit attempt.[74] Therefore, smokers with depression may respond better to smoking cessation interventions augmented with mood management techniques. Our results support this hypothesis. Pooled results from our meta-analysis demonstrate a small, positive effect of adding behavioral mood management therapy to smoking cessation cotreatments. The number needed to treat with mood management therapy plus NRT or antidepressants is 12 persons to get 1 additional person to quit smoking for at least 6 months. The strength of evidence is moderate. Only six identified trials provided enough detail to assess cessation rates among smokers with depression. Moreover, we found significant heterogeneity in intensity of mood management therapy across studies, which may influence estimates of effectiveness.

All of the included antidepressant trials showed small, positive effects on smoking cessation, but a summary estimate of effect was not statistically significant. However, the strength of evidence for the lack of benefit for antidepressants as a smoking cessation aid for smokers with depression is low. Sample sizes were small and the number achieving cessation few, which limits precision of estimates of effects and our ability to detect statistically significant differences. Also, we were able to include only five trials, of which there was significant heterogeneity in antidepressant type. Only bupropion and nortriptyline have proven efficacy as smoking cessation pharmacotherapies.[36,76] Meta-analysis results show little smoking cessation benefit for selective serotonin reuptake inhibitors such as sertraline and fluoxetine in the general population of smokers.[36] Because results may differ by pharmacotherapy used, caution should be taken in applying our findings to other antidepressants that may be used to aid smokers with depression in quitting smoking.

Offering NRT to smokers with depression appears to have a small, positive effect on smoking cessation rates among depressed smokers. Cessation rates ranged from 14 to 22% in the three included studies that reported outcomes of 12 months or longer.[44,57,64] These cessation rates are higher than the 3 to 5% of smokers who successfully maintain quit attempts a year later without treatment aids[77] and are comparable to NRT quit rates in the general population of smokers.[35] Yet, long-term cessation rates were lower for patients with current depressive symptoms[57] than for those who are history positive for MDD[44] (14% versus 22%, respectively). Smokers with current depressive symptoms may have greater difficulty quitting due to more issues with nicotine withdrawal or worsening of depressive symptoms during a quit attempt.[78] Smokers with current depressive symptoms may need additional support to make and maintain a quit attempt. The strength of evidence for NRT use among smokers with depression is moderate. Data were sparse; we were able to include only four trials. However, studies were of good quality and reported consistent results.

STRENGTHS AND LIMITATIONS

Our systematic review has a number of strengths that are consistent with the QUORUM reporting statement and the AMSTAR quality assessment of systematic reviews. These include a protocol-driven approach, a comprehensive literature search of multiple electronic databases, double data abstraction, quality assessment of the primary studies, and appropriate methods for combining estimates of effect. Despite these strengths, our review has several limitations.

Foremost is that few RCTs exist that test smoking cessation interventions among smokers with depression. The paucity of literature has important implications for this evidence review. First, in order to make meaningful comparisons, we created broad intervention categories that used different types of counseling modes (e.g., group, individual) and pharmacotherapies. Within each category, there is considerable heterogeneity. For example, we identified few medication trials and fewer with the same type of medication. Ideally, we would have wanted to analyze trials by specific medications since treatment effects may vary within broad classes of medications.

Second, few trials recruited smokers with current depression. In fact, many trials excluded patients with current or recent histories of depression. Therefore, many reports based classifications of depression on self-reported screening criteria (e.g., CES-D, BDI) for significant depressive symptoms. Self-report scales may be measures of general emotional distress or negative affect rather than specific depressive symptoms. In primary care settings, a positive depression screen has a positive predictive value of $\leq 50\%$ for MDD.[79] Thus, our review contains heterogeneity among the group of subjects included in trials classified as depressed. To address this heterogeneity, our protocol specified a stratified analysis by type of depression (e.g., history of MDD, current depressive symptoms, current MDD), but there were too few trials in any intervention category to follow this planned approach. Also, time since last episode, chronicity of depression, and other important variations in depressive disorders may be associated with outcomes. For example, some evidence supports that those with recurrent MDD compared to a single episode have worse outcomes[6] and may differentially respond to certain interventions that target their depressive symptoms during a quit attempt. Our review is unable to address this issue. Moreover, most studies included in this report excluded participants with comorbid alcohol or substance abuse. Results are likely not generalizable to groups with these comorbidities.

In many instances, we examined subgroup data for this evidence review. Including studies that reported on subgroups of individuals with depression has limitations. By doing so, we introduce the possibility of false-negative studies because many of these studies were not powered to detect clinically important treatment effects in depressed subgroups. Meta-analysis helps to address this limitation, but with relatively few studies of small sample sizes, our analyses may remain underpowered. In addition, subgroup analyses, unless specified a priori and part of a limited number of subgroups evaluated, may produce false-positive or spurious results.[80]

Data were limited on the majority of our key questions. No studies tested differential effects of smoking cessation interventions by treatment sequencing among smokers with depression. Literature on treatment differences by gender and depression status was also sparse. Our results on adverse effects are limited as well. Ideally, we would have conducted a separate search for adverse effects in the observational literature. However, it is unlikely that much literature exists on these types of interventions specific to our population of interest—smokers with a history of depression or with current depression. Lastly, few of the trials in this evidence review included VA users. Although veterans have higher rates of depression and smoking compared to the general population,[8-12] results should be generalizable to the VA population.

CONCLUSIONS

We identified only 16 trials, encompassing 1756 smokers with depression. Just three of these trials actively recruited participants with elevated depressive symptoms.[57,58,67] Most patients included in this review were history positive for depression; findings best apply to this population. For patients with current depression, we have little data. We were able to conduct meta-analyses of only two contrasts: (1) addition of any type of antidepressant and (2) treatment augmented by behavioral mood management counseling. Results of this systematic review indicate promising smoking cessation strategies for smokers with depression.

Table 11 summarizes the strength of evidence for each of our key questions and contrasts. Our results support a small, positive effect for adding mood management counseling for smoking cessation among patients with depression. However, it is uncertain if the effects of mood management counseling may differ by therapy mode (individual versus group therapy). We did not find adequate support for adding antidepressants; we may be underpowered to detect statistically significant differences. Evidence suggests support for adding NRT; however, included trials were too varied to be analyzed quantitatively. While most trials included in this evidence review were of good quality and had consistent results, data were sparse. We expect that future research will likely have an important impact on our confidence in the estimates of effectiveness of smoking cessation treatments for smokers with depression. However, evidence suggests that depression does not need to be resolved before tobacco cessation treatment is initiated. Smokers with depression can successfully maintain smoking cessation. To improve the likelihood of success, health care providers should consider encouraging their depressed patients who smoke to seek smoking cessation services that include behavioral mood management treatment and NRT.

Table 11. Summary of the Strength of Evidence for Key Questions 1 to 5

Number of studies (subjects)[a]	Domains pertaining to strength of evidence				Magnitude of effect and strength of evidence
	Risk of Bias: Design/ Quality	Consistency	Directness	Precision	Percentage abstinent from smoking at least 6 months postrandomization or relative risk ratio
Key Question 1: NRT					**Moderate SOE**
Moderate SOE	4 (699) RCT/ Good	Consistent	Direct	Imprecise	14 to 22%
Key Question 1: Antidepressant therapy					**Low SOE**
5 (484)	RCT/Good	Consistent	Direct	Imprecise	1.48 (95% CI 0.86 to 2.54)b
Key Question 1: Mood management treatment					**Moderate SOE**
6 (466)	RCT/Good	Consistent	Direct	Imprecise	1.45 (95% CI 1.01 to 2.07)c
Key Question 1: Other intervention strategies					**Low SOE**
3 (202)	RCT/ Fair	Inconsistent	Direct	Imprecise	17 to 39%
Key Question 2: Differential effects by depression status					**Insufficient SOE**
2 (305)	RCT/ Good	Inconsistent	Direct	Imprecise	18 to 39%
Key Question 3: Differential effects by gender					**Insufficient SOE**
1 (36)	RCT/ Good	Consistent	Direct	Imprecise	22%
Key Question 4: Differential effects by treatments delivered concurrently or sequentially					Insufficient SOE
0 (0)	---	---	---	---	---
Key Question 5: Adverse effects					**Insufficient SOE**
5 (1,652)	RCT/ Good	Inconsistent	Indirect	Imprecise	

[a] Numbers reflect participants with depression only for KQs 1 to 4 and all study participants for KQ 5.

[b] Magnitude of effect calculated from 3 trials included in meta-analysis (n = 255).

[c] Magnitude of effect calculated from 5 trials included in meta-analysis (n = 402).

Abbreviations: CI = confidence interval, RCT = randomized controlled trial, SOE = strength of evidence

FUTURE RESEARCH

While this review provides some evidence about smoking cessation strategies for patients with depression, more work is needed in this area. First, we found very little trial data on intervening with smokers who are currently depressed. Persons with depression are about twice as likely to be smokers than persons without depression.[5] Moreover, smokers with depression may experience more challenges when trying to make and maintain a quit attempt, such as greater negative mood symptoms from withdrawal, higher nicotine dependence, and greater likelihood of relapse, than smokers without depression.[17,18,21,22,24,81] Secondary analysis of existing smoking cessation trial data could advance our understanding of smoking cessation strategies for patients with depression. Future studies should be designed to test smoking cessation interventions for this vulnerable population. Next, within the trials we identified, we found little research on key moderators that may influence treatment effectiveness (e.g., gender, depression status). Moderator analysis will facilitate subgroup identification, which may lead to better treatment matching.[6]

Evidence is growing that combination pharmacotherapy is effective for the general population of smokers.[82] In 2009, the VA Pharmacy Benefits Management (PBM) Services released recommendations for the use of combination pharmacotherapy for tobacco use cessation. The VA PBM recommends combination NRT that involves the use of a longer acting NRT such as the patch in conjunction with a short-acting NRT (e.g., gum, inhaler, nasal spray) (http://www.pbm.va.gov). Future studies should be designed to allow for direct comparisons between combinations of likely efficacious NRT therapies for smokers with depression. Also, it is not known how to combine depression and smoking pharmacotherapies. Take, for example, a patient with depression who is improving on sertraline but wants to stop smoking. Should the provider add bupropion or change from sertraline to bupropion, which may risk worsening of depression? Future trials should investigate combination smoking cessation and depression pharmacotherapy among smokers with depression.

Behavioral counseling plus pharmacotherapy is considered the gold standard of care for effective smoking cessation interventions.[29,37,39] Smokers with psychiatric comorbidities may benefit from combined behavioral counseling and pharmacotherapy with longer therapeutic approaches (i.e., exceeding 8 to 12 weeks) to reduce likelihood of dropout and depression relapse.[41] Thus, future research should be designed to optimize dose, duration, and frequency of both behavioral counseling and pharmacotherapies. In addition, it is likely that patients with depression need strategies that target both depressive symptoms and smoking. Future research should seek to answer questions about the optimal sequencing of depression and smoking treatment content of smoking cessation interventions. Moreover, we were unable to tease apart the active components of individual therapies. Thus, important issues, such as mode of therapy (e.g., individual, group, telephone) and key therapeutic components (e.g., goal setting, monitoring of thoughts and moods, social support), cannot be answered by this systematic review. Future studies should be designed to disentangle active ingredients of behavioral counseling and the effects of delivery channels. Beyond scanning the reports included in this review, no attempt was made to synthesize information about adverse effects from observational studies and other data sources. Future research should be conducted to characterize adverse effects of treatment, including changes in negative affect and depressive symptoms.

REFERENCES

1. Danaei G, Ding EL, Mozaffarian D, et al. The preventable causes of death in the United States: comparative risk assessment of dietary, lifestyle, and metabolic risk factors. PLoS Med 2009;6(4):e1000058.

2. Mokdad AH, Marks JS, Stroup DF, et al. Actual causes of death in the United States, 2000. JAMA 2004;291(10):1238-45.

3. Cigarette smoking among adults--United States, 2006. MMWR Morb Mortal Wkly Rep 2007;56(44):1157-61.

4. Grant BF, Hasin DS, Chou SP, et al. Nicotine dependence and psychiatric disorders in the United States: results from the national epidemiologic survey on alcohol and related conditions. Arch Gen Psychiatry 2004;61(11):1107-15.

5. Lasser K, Boyd JW, Woolhandler S, et al. Smoking and mental illness: A population-based prevalence study. JAMA 2000;284(20):2606-10.

6. Ziedonis D, Hitsman B, Beckham JC, et al. Tobacco use and cessation in psychiatric disorders: National Institute of Mental Health report. Nicotine Tob Res 2008;10(12):1691-715.

7. Hall SM, Prochaska JJ. Treatment of smokers with co-occurring disorders: emphasis on integration in mental health and addiction treatment settings. Annu Rev Clin Psychol 2009;5:409-31.

8. Hamlett-Berry K, Davison J, Kivlahan DR, et al. Evidence-based national initiatives to address tobacco use as a public health priority in the Veterans Health Administration. Mil Med 2009;174(1):29-34.

9. Black DW, Carney CP, Forman-Hoffman VL, et al. Depression in veterans of the first Gulf War and comparable military controls. Ann Clin Psychiatry 2004;16(2):53-61.

10. Institute of Medicine. *Combating tobacco use in the military and veteran populations* Washington, DC: The National Academies Press 2009.

11. Fiedler N, Ozakinci G, Hallman W, et al. Military deployment to the Gulf War as a risk factor for psychiatric illness among US troops. Br J Psychiatry 2006;188:453-9.

12. Desai MM, Rosenheck RA, Craig TJ. Case-finding for depression among medical outpatients in the Veterans Health Administration. Med Care 2006;44(2):175-81.

13. Currie SR, Hodgins DC, el-Guebaly N, et al. Influence of depression and gender on smoking expectancies and temptations in alcoholics in early recovery. J Subst Abuse 2001;13(4):443-58.

14. Ischaki E, Gratziou C. Smoking and depression: Is smoking cessation effective? Ther Adv Respir Dis 2009;3(1):31-8.

15.   Berlin I, Covey LS. Pre-cessation depressive mood predicts failure to quit smoking: the role of coping and personality traits. Addiction 2006;101(12):1814-21.

16.   Breslau N, Johnson EO. Predicting smoking cessation and major depression in nicotine-dependent smokers. Am J Public Health 2000;90(7):1122-7.

17.   Kenney BA, Holahan CJ, Holahan CK, et al. Depressive symptoms, drinking problems, and smoking cessation in older smokers. Addict Behav 2009;34(6-7):548-53.

18.   Cinciripini PM, Wetter DW, Fouladi RT, et al. The effects of depressed mood on smoking cessation: mediation by postcessation self-efficacy. J Consult Clin Psychol 2003;71(2):292-301.

19.   Wiesbeck GA, Kuhl HC, Yaldizli O, et al. Tobacco smoking and depression--results from the WHO/ISBRA study. Neuropsychobiology 2008;57(1-2):26-31.

20.   Kinnunen T, Haukkala A, Korhonen T, et al. Depression and smoking across 25 years of the Normative Aging. Int J Psychiatry Med 2006;36(4):413-26.

21.   Glassman AH, Covey LS, Stetner F, et al. Smoking cessation and the course of major depression: a follow-up study. Lancet 2001;357(9272):1929-32.

22.   Niaura R, Britt DM, Shadel WG, et al. Symptoms of depression and survival experience among three samples of smokers trying to quit. Psychol Addict Behav 2001;15(1):13-7.

23.   Pomerleau CS, Zucker AN, Stewart AJ. Characterizing concerns about post-cessation weight gain: Results from a national survey of women smokers. Nicotine Tob Res 2001;3(1):51-60.

24.   Tsoh JY, Humfleet GL, Munoz RF, et al. Development of major depression after treatment for smoking cessation. Am J Psychiatry 2000;157(3):368-74.

25.   Siru R, Hulse GK, Tait RJ. Assessing motivation to quit smoking in people with mental illness: a review. Addiction 2009;104(5):719-33.

26.   Prochaska JJ, Rossi JS, Redding CA, et al. Depressed smokers and stage of change: implications for treatment interventions. Drug Alcohol Depend 2004;76(2):143-51.

27.   Hitsman B, Moss TG, Montoya ID, et al. Treatment of tobacco dependence in mental health and addictive disorders. Can J Psychiatry 2009;54(6):368-78.

28.   Hall SM. Nicotine interventions with comorbid populations. Am J Prev Med 2007;33(6 Suppl):S406-13.

29.   Stead LF, Perera R, Lancaster T. Telephone counselling for smoking cessation. Cochrane Database Syst Rev 2006;3:CD002850.

30.   Shiffman S, Ferguson SG. Nicotine patch therapy prior to quitting smoking: a meta-analysis. Addiction 2008;103(4):557-63.

31.   Baddoura R, Wehbeh-Chidiac C. Prevalence of tobacco use among the adult Lebanese population. East Mediterr Health J 2001;7(4-5):819-28.

32.   Stead LF, Bergson G, Lancaster T. Physician advice for smoking cessation. Cochrane Database Syst Rev 2008(2):CD000165.

33.   Lancaster T, Stead LF. Individual behavioural counselling for smoking cessation. Cochrane Database Syst Rev 2005(2):CD001292.

34.   Stead LF, Lancaster T. Group behaviour therapy programmes for smoking cessation. Cochrane Database Syst Rev 2005(2):CD001007.

35.   Stead LF, Perera R, Bullen C, et al. Nicotine replacement therapy for smoking cessation. Cochrane Database Syst Rev 2008(1):CD000146.

36.   Hughes JR, Stead LF, Lancaster T. Antidepressants for smoking cessation. Cochrane Database Syst Rev 2007(1):CD000031.

37.   Fiore MC, Jaén CR, Baker TB, et al. Treating Tobacco Use and Dependence: 2008 Update. Quick Reference Guide for Clinicians. Rockville, MD: US Department of Health and Human Services. Public Health Service. April 2009. Available at: http://www.ahrq.gov/clinic/tobacco/tobaqrg.pdf. Accessed November 2010.

38.   Rabius V, Pike KJ, Hunter J, et al. Effects of frequency and duration in telephone counselling for smoking cessation. Tob Control 2007;16 Suppl 1:i71-4.

39.   An LC, Zhu SH, Nelson DB, et al. Benefits of telephone care over primary care for smoking cessation: a randomized trial. Arch Intern Med 2006;166(5):536-42.

40.   Weinberger AH, Maciejewski PK, McKee SA, et al. Gender differences in associations between lifetime alcohol, depression, panic disorder, and posttraumatic stress disorder and tobacco withdrawal. Am J Addict 2009;18(2):140-7.

41.   Gelenberg AJ, de Leon J, Evins AE, et al. Smoking cessation in patients with psychiatric disorders. Prim Care Companion J Clin Psychiatry 2008;10(1):52-8.

42.   Agency for Healthcare Research and Quality. Methods Guide for Effectiveness and Comparative Effectiveness Reviews. Rockville, MD: Agency for Healthcare Research and Quality. Available at: http://www.effectivehealthcare.ahrq.gov/index.cfm/search-for-guides-reviews-and-reports/?pageaction=displayproduct&productid=318. Accessed November 11, 2010.

43.   West R, Hajek P, Stead L, et al. Outcome criteria in smoking cessation trials: proposal for a common standard. Addiction 2005;100(3):299-303.

44.   Hall SM, Munoz RF, Reus VI, et al. Mood management and nicotine gum in smoking treatment: a therapeutic contact and placebo-controlled study. J Consult Clin Psychol 1996;64(5):1003-9.

45. Hall SM, Reus VI, Munoz RF, et al. Nortriptyline and cognitive-behavioral therapy in the treatment of cigarette smoking. Arch Gen Psychiatry 1998;55(8):683-90.

46. Cochran WG. The Combination of Estimates from Different Experiments. Biometrics 1954;10(1):101-129.

47. Fleiss JL. Analysis of data from multiclinic trials. Control Clin Trials 1986;7(4):267-75.

48. Higgins JP, Thompson SG. Quantifying heterogeneity in a meta-analysis. Stat Med 2002;21(11):1539-58.

49. Higgins JP, Greenberg S. Cochrane Handbook for Systematic Reviews of Interventions Version 5.0.2 [updated September 2009]. The Cochrane Collaboration, 2009. Available from www.cochrane-handbook.org.

50. Atkins D, Best D, Briss PA, et al. Grading quality of evidence and strength of recommendations. BMJ 2004;328(7454):1490.

51. Munoz RF, Marin BV, Posner SF, et al. Mood management mail intervention increases abstinence rates for Spanish-speaking Latino smokers. Am J Community Psychol 1997;25(3):325-43.

52. Kinnunen T, Doherty K, Militello FS, et al. Depression and smoking cessation: characteristics of depressed smokers and effects of nicotine replacement. J Consult Clin Psychol 1996;64(4):791-8.

53. Brown RA, Kahler CW, Niaura R, et al. Cognitive-behavioral treatment for depression in smoking cessation. J Consult Clin Psychol 2001;69(3):471-80.

54. Covey LS, Glassman AH, Stetner F, et al. A randomized trial of sertraline as a cessation aid for smokers with a history of major depression. Am J Psychiatry 2002;159(10):1731-7.

55. Evins AE, Culhane MA, Alpert JE, et al. A controlled trial of bupropion added to nicotine patch and behavioral therapy for smoking cessation in adults with unipolar depressive disorders. J Clin Psychopharmacol 2008;28(6):660-6.

56. Vickers KS, Patten CA, Lewis BA, et al. Feasibility of an exercise counseling intervention for depressed women smokers. Nicotine Tob Res 2009;11(8):985-95.

57. Hall SM, Tsoh JY, Prochaska JJ, et al. Treatment for cigarette smoking among depressed mental health outpatients: a randomized clinical trial. Am J Public Health 2006;96(10):1808-14.

58. MacPherson L, Tull MT, Matusiewicz AK, et al. Randomized controlled trial of behavioral activation smoking cessation treatment for smokers with elevated eepressive symptoms. J Consult Clin Psychol 2010;78(1):55-61.

59. Duffy SA, Ronis DL, Valenstein M, et al. A tailored smoking, alcohol, and depression intervention for head and neck cancer patients. Cancer Epidemiol Biomarkers Prev 2006;15(11):2203-8.

60. Hall SM, Munoz RF, Reus VI. Cognitive-behavioral intervention increases abstinence rates for depressive-history smokers. J Consult Clin Psychol 1994;62(1):141-6.

61. Hayford KE, Patten CA, Rummans TA, et al. Efficacy of bupropion for smoking cessation in smokers with a former history of major depression or alcoholism. Br J Psychiatry 1999;174:173-8.

62. Saules KK, Schuh LM, Arfken CL, et al. Double-blind placebo-controlled trial of fluoxetine in smoking cessation treatment including nicotine patch and cognitive-behavioral group therapy. Am J Addict 2004;13(5):438-46.

63. Covey LS, Glassman AH, Stetner F. Naltrexone effects on short-term and long-term smoking cessation. J Addict Dis 1999;18(1):31-40.

64. Kinnunen T, Korhonen T, Garvey AJ. Role of nicotine gum and pretreatment depressive symptoms in smoking cessation: twelve-month results of a randomized placebo controlled trial. Int J Psychiatry Med 2008;38(3):373-89.

65. Katon WJ. Clinical and health services relationships between major depression, depressive symptoms, and general medical illness. Biol Psychiatry 2003;54(3):216-26.

66. John U, Meyer C, Rumpf HJ, et al. Depressive disorders are related to nicotine dependence in the population but do not necessarily hamper smoking cessation. J Clin Psychiatry 2004;65(2):169-76.

67. Vickers KS, Patten CA, Clark MM, et al. Exercise intervention for women with depressive symptoms interested in smoking cessation. *Society for Research on Nicotine and Tobacco 11th Annual Meeting 20-23 March 2005; Prague, Czech Republic*; 2005.

68. Nides M, Glover ED, Reus VI, et al. Varenicline versus bupropion SR or placebo for smoking cessation: a pooled analysis. Am J Health Behav 2008;32(6):664-75.

69. Nides M. Update on Pharmacologic Options for Smoking Cessation Treatment. Am J Med 2008;121(4 SUPPL.):S20-S31.

70. Campbell AR, Anderson KD. Mental health stability in veterans with posttraumatic stress disorder receiving varenicline. Am J Health Syst Pharm 2010;67(21):1832-7.

71. Haaga DA, Thorndike FP, Friedman-Wheeler DG, et al. Cognitive coping skills and depression vulnerability among cigarette smokers. Addict Behav 2004;29(6):1109-22.

72. Kahler CW, Brown RA, Ramsey SE, et al. Negative mood, depressive symptoms, and major depression after smoking cessation treatment in smokers with a history of major depressive disorder. J Abnorm Psychol 2002;111(4):670-5.

73.   Kahler CW, Brown RA, Strong DR, et al. History of major depressive disorder among smokers in cessation treatment: associations with dysfunctional attitudes and coping. Addict Behav 2003;28(6):1033-47.

74.   Carmody TP. Affect regulation, nicotine addiction, and smoking cessation. J Psychoactive Drugs 1992;24(2):111-22.

75.   Hall SM, Munoz RF, Reus VI, et al. Nicotine, negative affect, and depression. J Consult Clin Psychol 1993;61(5):761-7.

76.   Hurt RD, Sachs DP, Glover ED, et al. A comparison of sustained-release bupropion and placebo for smoking cessation. N Engl J Med 1997;337(17):1195-202.

77.   Hughes JR, Keely J, Naud S. Shape of the relapse curve and long-term abstinence among untreated smokers. Addiction 2004;99(1):29-38.

78.   Haas AL, Munoz RF, Humfleet GL, et al. Influences of mood, depression history, and treatment modality on outcomes in smoking cessation. J Consult Clin Psychol 2004;72(4):563-70.

79.   Williams JW, Jr., Pignone M, Ramirez G, et al. Identifying depression in primary care: a literature synthesis of case-finding instruments. Gen Hosp Psychiatry 2002;24(4):225-37.

80.   Sun X, Briel M, Walter SD, et al. Is a subgroup effect believable? Updating criteria to evaluate the credibility of subgroup analyses. BMJ 2010;340:c117.

81.   Pomerleau CS, Brouwer RJ, Pomerleau OF. Emergence of depression during early abstinence in depressed and non-depressed women smokers. J Addict Dis 2001;20(1):73-80.

82.   Shah SD, Wilken LA, Winkler SR, et al. Systematic review and meta-analysis of combination therapy for smoking cessation. J Am Pharm Assoc (2003) 2008;48(5):659-65.

APPENDIX A: SEARCH STRATEGY

PubMed: Search on March 10, 2010 (yield = 463 articles)

(("smoking cessation"[MeSH Terms] OR ("smoking"[All Fields] AND "cessation"[All Fields]) OR "smoking cessation"[All Fields]) OR ("Smoking/prevention and control"[Mesh:noexp] OR "Smoking/therapy"[Mesh:noexp])) AND ("Depression"[Mesh] OR (("Depressive Disorder"[Mesh:noexp] OR "Depressive Disorder, Major"[Mesh]) OR "Dysthymic Disorder"[Mesh]))

Embase: Search on March 10, 2010 (yield = 489)

'depression'/de OR 'agitated depression'/exp OR 'atypical depression'/exp OR 'depressive psychosis'/exp OR 'dysphoria'/exp OR 'dysthymia'/exp OR 'endogenous depression'/exp OR 'major depression'/exp OR 'masked depression'/exp OR 'melancholia'/exp OR 'mixed anxiety and depression'/exp OR 'mixed depression and dementia'/exp OR 'mourning syndrome'/exp OR 'organic depression'/exp OR 'reactive depression'/exp OR 'recurrent brief depression'/exp AND ('smoking cessation'/exp/mj OR 'smoking cessation program'/exp/mj)

PsycINFO: Search on March 10, 2010 (yield = 219)

(DE "Depression (Emotion)") or (DE "Major Depression" or DE "Affective Disorders" or DE "Anaclitic Depression" or DE "Dysthymic Disorder" or DE "Endogenous Depression" or DE "Reactive Depression" or DE "Recurrent Depression" or DE "Treatment Resistant Depression") and (("Smoking Cessation" or (DE "Drug Rehabilitation") and (DE "Tobacco Smoking"))

Cochrane Library: Search on March 10, 2010 (yield = 169)

Smoking cessation and depression (limit clinical trials)

APPENDIX B: REVIEWER COMMENTS AND RESPONSES

Reviewer	Comment	Response
Question 1: Are the objectives, scope, and methods for this review clearly described?		
1	Yes – no comment	Thank you.
2	Yes – excellent review and very clearly written	Thank you.
3	The selection of appropriate outcome measures warrants more attention on p 14 or p 17 line 8. See the Hughes et al 2003 report of recommendations of the abstinence outcome measures work-group of the Society for Research on Nicotine and Tobacco (Hughes J. R., Keely J. P., Niaura R. S., Ossip-Klein D. J., Richmond R. L., Swan G. E. Measures of abstinence in clinical trials: issues and recommendations. *Nicotine Tob Res* 2003; **5**: 13–25).	We have further clarified outcome measures in the methods section. Operationalization of smoking cessation was informed by those used in Cochrane reviews of smoking cessation which is based on the Russel Standard (West R, Hajek P, Stead L, Stapleton J. Outcome criteria in smoking cessation trials: proposal for a common standard. *Addiction* 2005;100(3):299-303).
	The availability of biological verification of self-report (CO or cotinine) in only a couple of studies should also be noted as a limitation in this literature.	All included studies use biological verification of self-report smoking cessation.
	The systematic search strategy is among the many strengths of the review. It may be implicit in the MESH term "smoking", but it would be worth indicating on p 13 and/or in Appendix A that "nicotine" and "tobacco" are subsumed in that category. Tobacco currently only appears under PsycINFO.	"Tobacco" and "nicotine" are not indexed under the MESH term "smoking." Adding these terms yields an additional 81 articles of which none met our eligibility criteria.
4	Yes – no comment	Thank you.
5	Yes – no comment	Thank you.
6	Yes - Thanks for the opportunity to see this work. The key questions are succinctly and clearly defined in logical sequence. Language is clear and concise. Figure 1 page 13 is helpful. In general I think this review has been well conducted and well summarized.	Thank you.
Question 2: Is there any indication of bias in our synthesis of the evidence?		
1	No – no comment	Thank you.
2	P 25 lines 22-23----check numbers	Numbers are correct.
	P 27 line 11----it would be easier for the reader if you consistently describe the comparisons being made. For example, it would be a lot easier to grasp this if the subtitle was: "Antidepressant therapy +cotreatment versus placebo +co-treatment" rather than how it is written. Same issue occurs again in line 15---I would switch "antidepressants" and "behavioral"	We agree and have made the changes requested.
	P 29 line 15 table 7--add in risk estimates	Comparisons nonsignificant and risk estimates not reported.
3	No - Comments: The report appears to be rigorously objective.	Thank you.
4	No – no comment	Acknowledged

Reviewer	Comment	Response
5	No – no comment	Acknowledged
6	Possibly - Search: Limiting the search to English Language only will introduce bias, as will limiting the search to only the peer reviewed literature (publication bias). There may be other important trials in progress.	Non-English language articles are beyond the scope of this review. Inclusion of non–peer reviewed literature is controversial as these reports are often incomplete and can differ from final peer reviewed publication. An advantage of non-peer reviewed literature is a greater ability to detect publication bias. For this review, we thought the potential negatives of included these types of reports outweighed the potential advantages.
	Page 4: when referring to small positive effects of trials it is unclear whether these are statistically or clinically important differences? Did they "show" effects? Or simply "suggest" effects? Or just "trends" that could be due to chance. Could the wording here be tightened so this is clearer?	We have added greater specificity to the language.
	Page14: it is unclear why hospital based interventions were excluded? If seeking to include trials of people with current depressive symptoms, then an inpatient setting might capture some of these? (key question 2) Ditto the exclusion of relapse prevention trials may have excluded some direct or indirect evidence of efficacy of sequential treatment strategies (key question 4)	Stakeholders interested in outpatients and smoking cessation. However, we agree that including studies of relapse prevention could yield some indirect evidence but we thought that this would be too indirect for our purposes in this review.
Question 3: Are there any studies on of interest to the VA that we have overlooked?		
1	NO- no comment	Acknowledged
2	No – no comment	Acknowledged
3	The following study by McClure et al. appears to meet the criteria in Table 1 and is of particular interest to VHA given the focus on varenicline. If there is a reason for exclusion it would be important to clarify and there would still appear to be value in addressing the findings as they relate to KQ5 since there is currently no mention of varenicline in the document. McClure JB, Swan GE, Jack L, Catz SL, Zbikowski SM, McAfee TA, Deprey M, Richards J, Javitz H, Mood, side-effects and smoking outcomes among persons with and without probable lifetime depression taking varenicline. J Gen Intern Med. 2009 May;24(5):563-9. Epub 2009 Feb 24.	We identified and excluded McClure study because report did not provide data on rates of smoking cessation for the depressed subgroup by intervention arm. Therefore, we could not include these data in our analysis of the comparative effectiveness of smoking cessation interventions for depressed patients.
	Two recent qualitative reviews also seem worth citing in the background: Hitsman B, Moss TG, Montoya ID, George TP. Treatment of tobacco dependence in mental health and addictive disorders. Can J Psychiatry. 2009 Jun;54(6):368-78. Review. Hall SM. Nicotine interventions with comorbid populations. Am J Prev Med. 2007 Dec;33(6 Suppl):S406-13.	Thank you for this suggestion. We have added these to the background section.
4	No – no comment	Acknowledged
5	No – no comment	Acknowledged

Reviewer	Comment	Response
6	Excluding evidence based on timing of outcome reporting; figure 2 page 20. I have trouble reconciling what I read in the report results with what is detailed about trial flow in figure 2. Figure 2 suggests trials were excluded based on their choice of outcomes, or their choice of outcome reporting timepoint post intervention. In general terms, excluding evidence on the basis of outcomes is not recommended, if the trials otherwise meet inclusion criteria (population, design, intervention). For the 6 articles that reported outcomes of interest, but not at 6 and 12 months, it is possible that useful data do exist – but not in the published reports. Some description of these trials and their data might be informative, even if they are not subsequently able to contribute to predefined meta-analyses, or be used to inform the evidence summary. This is also true for the 14 articles that did not report the outcome of interest in their publications but otherwise met inclusion criteria (design, population, intervention) – perhaps the outcome data you sought does exist, and might be available from investigators.	As we described, few (n = 3) of the studies enrolled patients with depressive symptoms. Most included studies are secondary analysis, using history of depression. The studies excluded typically report smoking cessation outcomes, but not in the subgroup of interest (those with depression) and many are small without the power to evaluate interaction effects between depression and smoking cessation interventions. Also 6- and 12-month outcomes are clinically relevant. Contacting the authors for additional data is beyond the scope of these reviews. However, we've raised the possibility of missing studies with unpublished but relevant outcomes.
	In summarizing evidence, and if making suggestions for a future research agenda, then acknowledging these additional trials might be helpful: rather than undertaking new trials, considering making better use of existing data is also important. This can take the form of secondary analyses of existing trial data, or attempting individual patient data meta-analysis	The suggestions for patient level meta-analysis or secondary analysis of existing trial data has been incorporated into possibilities for future research.
Question 4: Please write additional suggestions or comments below. If applicable, please indicate the page and line numbers from the draft report.		
1	Comments were about the topic in general and not the report.	OK

Comparative Effectiveness of Smoking Cessation Treatments for Patients With Depression

Reviewer	Comment	Response
2	P1 line 5---add prevalence	We added prevalence.
	P3 line 12---do you include chantix?	Yes, but no trials using this drug met our eligibility criteria.
	P4 line 15---clarify what the antidepressant trials are compared to	We have clarified in text.
	P 5 line 10 ---clarify: does "control condition" belong in this sentence	Yes it does.
	P 6 line 6---I would rephrase this "…does treatment effectiveness differ by whether smoking cessation/depression treatments are delivered concurrently or sequentially?"	We have made this change.
	P 8 line 12---"for adding behavioral mood management counseling to ____ what?	We have clarified in text.
	P 10 line 14-16--- clarify the sequential/concurrent text. perhaps add an example on line 16. "… depression. For example…".	We have clarified in text.
	P 10 line 12 ---might add sentence after "sequentially" that says, "It is plausible but unstudied" if this is true.	We have added this sentence.
	P 19 line 7---? Manually pulled? You might rephrase this	We have rephrased this sentence.
	P 21 table 3---I think you should try and fit this on one page and definitely should add the setting to this table. Please also define FTND	We have modified table and "FTND" is defined in the footnotes of Table 3.
	P 27 line 22 table---note it should be "approach" not "approached". It would be nice to include a summary estimate in this table as well as many of the others also.	We have made this change and include summary estimates in the text, when available, for the comparisons of interest, smokers with depression by intervention arm.
	P 28 line 10---switch antidepressant and behavioral to make the comparisons clearer	We have changed all the title to make this clearer.
	P 29 line 15 table 7--add in risk estimates	We include risk estimates in the text, when available, for the comparisons of interest, smokers with depression by intervention arm.
	P 29, line 23---clarify what active control is	We have added example of active control.
	p 32 line 9 use "at" rather than "of"	We have made this change.
	Table 9---risk estimates would be helpful	We include risk estimates in the text, when available, for the comparisons of interest, smokers with depression.
	39 line 18---intervention rather than "interventions"	We have made this change.
	P 40. I would move the full sentence beginning in line 11-12 to the beginning of the paragraph	We respectfully disagree. This sentence belongs in the paragraph about mood management treatments.
	P 44 line 19---??? "can make"????	We have clarified the language.

Reviewer	Comment	Response
3	Varenicline is not mentioned in the document. Perhaps the basis for the McClure et al (2009) trial analysis was not evident to me for KQs 1-4, but the data on adverse effects seem highly relevant to Key Question 5 and use of varenicline for patients with MH diagnoses is of high interest within VHA, including recently revised criteria for use that emphasize psychiatric stability.	We did not exclude trials that used varenicline. No trials using varenicline met our eligibility criteria. Therefore, it is beyond the scope of this report to discuss adverse effects for therapies not included in included trials. We, however, now briefly discuss use of varenicline for veteran with mental health issues in the discussion section.
	The report should be more explicit in distinguishing history of depression from current depression that met diagnostic criteria and from current depression symptoms based on exceeding assessment thresholds. The identified language convention in p 23 line 11-13 does not seem to be applied consistently and it combines current depressive symptoms with current depression diagnosis. Similarly, on P 3 line 21 – among 3 studies that recruited participants with current depression, did some require that participants meet diagnostic criteria and others use assessments in the absence of diagnoses? Other statements to clarify history vs. current vs. either are p 25 line 7; p 29 line 23, p 30 line 6, p 30 line 11, p 31 line 20, p 40 line 14, Table 10 footnote b. Consider adding a footnote to Table 3 to designate the distinct meanings of current depression.	The reviewer is correct that we combined current and history-positive studies. As outlined in our research questions, we assessed the comparative effectiveness of smoking cessation strategies of patients with a history of a depressive disorder or current significant depressive symptoms. We, however, planned a priori to conduct subgroup analyses by depression status but were unable to do so due to low number of studies per comparison. We note this as a limitation of our study

We state the method of depression assessment for the three studies that recruited participants with current depression or elevated depressive symptoms on page 23 lines 9-12. We have clarified footnote b of table 10. |
	Regarding Key Question 2, the dimension at issue appears to be recency (i.e., history vs. current) or "type" (p 42 lines 19-20). Severity per se can vary widely among those classified as currently depressed, but this was not reflected in analyses.	For Key Question 2, we were interested in depression status at time entering trial. This could be operationalized as type or symptom severity at study entry. No studies conducted subgroup or interaction effects based on symptom severity at study entry. Therefore, we only reported on two studies that identified results based on depression type. For Key Question 2, we clarify that we were interested in depression status at study entry throughout the revised report. We intended to conduct subgroup analysis by depression status but number of studies was too few.
	RR is a conventional way to report trial outcomes, however to increase clinical relevance of effect sizes it would be helpful to report NNT or to advocate that this be included in future reports. For the Discussion, consider quantifying effects with NNT where possible (e.g., p 40 line 11).	According to the Cochrane Handbook, NNT cannot be combined for a summary estimate in meta-analysis. We, therefore use RR for our analyses. We, however, have computed a NNT for our significant summary effect for the addition of mood management treatments.
	As noted in the Discussion, most subgroup analyses warrant cautious interpretation. A recent reference at p 43 line 11 would help to emphasize that point (e.g., Sun X, Briel M, Walter SD, Guyatt GH. Is a subgroup effect believable? Updating criteria to evaluate the credibility of subgroup analyses. BMJ. 2010 Mar 30;340 doi: 10.1136/bmj.c117). It would also be useful to identify subgroup analyses reported in the selected studies as a priori or post hoc (e.g., p 5 line 20).	Thank you for the citation. We have added this to the report. Also studies did not state that subgroup analyses were conducted a priori and, thus, powered to detect interaction effects. We noted this as a limitation.

Reviewer	Comment	Response
3	Most of the studies excluded patients with current/recent substance use or substance use disorders. Given the high comorbidity of alcohol and other substance use disorders with smoking and depression, this is a limitation to generalizability worth noting.	We have added this as a limitation.
	There is evidence in the broader literature about the role of combination pharmacotherapy (e.g., combination NRT; see Shah SD, Wilken LA, Winkler SR, Lin SJ. Review and meta-analysis of combination therapy for smoking cessation. J Am Pharm Assoc (2003). 2008 Sep-Oct;48(5):659-65.) and this has resulted in guidance through VA Pharmacy Benefits (PBM-MAP Recommendations for Use of Combination Therapy in Tobacco Use Cessation; http://www.pbm.va.gov or http://vaww.pbm.va.gov) . This is an important area for future research on those with depression and is worth identifying in the Discussion and considering for the Executive Summary on p 7. This could also be cited on p 10 line 3 in the context of individual forms of NRT. P 39 line 20 should specify that the 4 trials involved single forms of NRT and none involved combinations. P 41 para 2 and p 46 last full sentence are other locations to raise this point.	We agree and stated this in our discussion of future research in and in the executive summary that combination therapies are an important area of future study. We have expanded this section and added VA PBM-specific information per the reviewer's suggestion. We also have clarified that the NRT trials are single-form NRT trials.
	KQ4 has high clinical relevance. Despite the absence of systematic analyses that address this issue, it would be useful to comment on whether/how current depression was addressed (e.g., with concurrent anti-depressants or psychotherapy) other than in conditions that involved mood management or bupropion, etc., and whether any anti-depressant doses were in the therapeutic range for treatment of depression (e.g., p 40 para 3). It seems important to comment on whether the evidence better addresses effects of smoking cessation in the context of treatment resistant depression or untreated depression (e.g., p 41 para 2 or p 42 para 2). The guidance on p 44 para 2 seems to suggest that behavioral mood management and NRT are adequate in the context of unresolved/untreated depression rather than encouraging concurrent patient engagement in guideline concordant care to address the depression. Note the contrast with the example on p 46 para 2 and p 47 first full sentence.	All but a few studies included in this report excluded MDD positive patients. Most patients included in this report could only be categorized as symptom positive, with no information on treatment resistance in the original papers. Therefore, we cannot comment on the effects of these smoking cessation strategies on patients with treatment resistant depression. Also we have clarified that we refer to the effects of antidepressants on smoking cessation. We were able to assess that antidepressant doses were in the therapeutic range. We have added this level of detail to the report.
	As noted on p 47, differential effects of mode of therapy could not be answered with available data. Since the issue of group vs. individual behavioral interventions has high relevance to implementation feasibility, it seems worth noting in regard to the heterogeneity of treatment categories (p 42 line 8). Uncertainty about advantages of individual vs. group modality for mood management (p 44 line 11) also would be useful to clarify.	We have added this clarification.
	Table 3 – recheck sample description for Duffy; p 63 indicated 69% with current depression?	Our numbers are correct. In Duffy et al., 69% of the total sample had depression but only 35% (n = 64) had comorbid depression and smoking at baseline.
4	In general, this report is thorough, well-written and objective. The reader gains a great deal of knowledge from the review of studies. Several specific comments are provided below. With the exception of the comment about exclusion of studies relating to Figure 2 on page 20, most of these comments are relatively trivial, but attention to them may slightly strengthen the review.	Thank you.

Reviewer	Comment	Response
4	On page 10, line 20, the meaning of the following sentence is a bit opaque. This sentence could perhaps be eliminated or rewritten: "Yet the extent to which level of depressive symptoms affects smoking cessation efforts has not yet been synthesized."	We agree and have deleted this sentence.
	On page 10, line 23 (going onto page 11), the sentence, "Treating depression first may lead to greater treatment adherence and, consequently, better cessation rates" while having face validity, represents speculation, and that point should be made clear here.	We agree and have clarified that this is plausible but not yet known.
	On page 11, line 2, likewise the sentence, "Smokers with psychiatric comorbidities may benefit from combined behavioral counseling and 3 pharmacotherapy with longer therapeutic smoking cessation approaches (i.e., exceeding 8 to 12 4 weeks) to reduce likelihood of dropout and depression relapse" while a reasonable supposition actually poses a hypothesis to be examined, but the language here does not make that point entirely clear.	The original language does not state this as a known. Our language states that these approaches *may* be beneficial. We then state that this needs to be studied.
	Page 14, line 10, Table 1: The exclusion for relapse prevention as an outcome is not entirely graspable. Does it mean that studies which randomized participants who had already quit and evaluated relapse as an outcome were excluded? If so, try to make this point clearer perhaps via an additional footnote.	We have added a footnote that defines relapse prevention.
	Page 20, Figure 2: 6 studies were excluded because the "Main outcome not reported at desired interval." However, the report gives no justification for the outcome intervals selected (self-reported 7 day abstinence at 6–12 months or [secondarily] abstinence at 3–4 months.) Considering that only 16 RCTs were ultimately included in the analysis, there must be more justification for the exclusion of 6 potential studies simply on the basis of outcome interval when we really do not know the optimal interval for testing abstinence that might predict long term quitting.	We have further clarified outcome measures in the methods section. Operationalization of smoking cessation was informed by those used in Cochrane reviews of smoking cessation which is based on the Russel Standard (West R, Hajek P, Stead L, Stapleton J. Outcome criteria in smoking cessation trials: proposal for a common standard. *Addiction* 2005;100(3):299-303). Also, the six excluded studies reported outcomes at end of treatment. End of treatment is not likely to be a good indicator of long-term smoking cessation.
	Page 24, line 11, "antidepressants" should be singular "antidepressant."	We have made this change.
	Page 24, lines 15-16, oral naltrexone should not be called "long acting." The parent drug has an average half-life of 4 hours, the active metabolite an average half-life of 12 hours. The way it is described here, it could be confused with the long acting injectable naltrexone which has therapeutic effects lasting 28 days.	The original paper refers to the naltrexone used in the study as "long acting." We have clarified that the trial used the pill form of naltrexone.
	Page 27, line 22, Table 6, second and third columns, second row, change "approached" to "approach."	We have made this change.

Reviewer	Comment	Response
4	Page 30, line 4, consider rewording the sentence, "Overall, we did not find enough evidence to support adding antidepressants to other smoking cessation cotreatments for persons with prior histories of depression." Most of the studies looked at participants with prior histories of depression. If the patient has current depression and is trying to quit, most likely we would want her/him on an antidepressant for its effects on depression regardless of its lack of effect for smoking cessation. The wording as is could leave the impression that these patients should not be on antidepressants at all.	Our primary outcome of interest was smoking cessation. Therefore, we were interested if adding antidepressants to smoking cessation cotreatments improves smoking cessation outcomes. It is an empirical question if persons with current depression undergoing a quit attempt receive relief from their depression with antidepressants therapy alone versus psychotherapy or combination psychotherapy and pharmacotherapy for depression. We, however, have reworded the sentence so that it is clear we are are referring to antidepressant effects on smoking cessation alone.
	Page 35, line 7, rewrite sentence, "Participants were randomized to 12 weeks of bupropion plus a cotreatment consisting of 8 weeks of transdermal NRT and 13 sessions of group CBT smoking cessation counseling or cotreatment plus placebo." One potential suggestion is: "Participants were randomized to 12 weeks of bupropion vs. placebo. Both groups received a cotreatment consisting of 8 weeks of transdermal NRT and 13 sessions of group CBT smoking cessation counseling.	We have changed the wording per the reviewer's suggestion.
	Page 35, line 9 creates some confusion by saying "Among participants who were history positive for unipolar depression . . ." Whereas, earlier on line 6, the text indicates that "Evins (2008) recruited 199 smokers who were history positive for unipolar depressive disorders." The text in line 9 makes it sound like all subjects were not history positive, but line 6 indicates that they were. It appears that the entire paragraph beginning on line 6 needs reworking.	We have revised the paragraph in order to better explain that Evins (2008) recruited participants with lifetime histories of unipolar depression but then assessed cessation rates by current versus history-positive groups.
	Page 36, lines 2–8, the differences in n's between men and women and the overall small sample size really preclude drawing any conclusions from these data. Please either supply the quit rates for men or comment that the small samples sizes render the study very inconclusive. A general caveat about this type of finding which occurs in other areas of the review appears on page 43, lines 5–11, but it also may be helpful to include such caveats in the specific areas of the report they pertain to. This strategy introduces redundancy but may aid clarity.	We agree with the reviewer that the small number of participants limits our ability to draw any conclusion. We state this as a global limitation of many of our findings. The study did not report quit rates for men beyond end of treatment assessments.
	Page 38, Table 10, if possible it would be good add a column listing the interventions. The interventions are listed in other tables, but it is difficult for the reader to flip back and forth. The clinical meaning of the adverse events is not too apparent if the reader is unsure of the intervention possibly related to the adverse events.	We have added a column describing the interventions.
	Page 40, lines 1–4, the wording here could give the reader the impression that the interventions mentioned are inefficacious, when, in fact, they have been insufficiently studied. An attempt to make that clear via the final clause in the paragraph does not quite get there. This point should be explicitly stated.	We have clarified that these are understudied strategies that need further examination.
	Page 40, line 6, the sentence, "Smokers with depression are more likely to have increased levels of negative precessation and postcessation" is poorly phrased. How about, "Smokers with depression are more likely to have increased levels of negative mood both pre- and post-cessation."	We have made this word change.

Reviewer	Comment	Response
4	Page 41, line 13, remove word "elevated."	We removed this word.
	Page 44, line 19, the sentence, "Smokers with depression can make and maintain smoking cessation" is a little awkward and would benefit from rewording.	We have reworded this sentence.
5	Overall, I found the report extremely clear and well-written. I learned a lot from the content, particularly how seldom this important topic has been adequately studied.	Thank you.
	Page 7, lines 11-14 – Which category would varenicline fit into? Also, I think it matters whether the antidepressant being studied is bupropion or nortriptyline (both endorsed by the PHS guidelines) vs. the other antidepressants. On the other hand, none of the antidepressant studies really showed much, so maybe it is not necessary to separate them out.	We had insufficient number of trials to assess antidepressant effects by specific drug. We state this as a limitation.
	Page 38 – I would change the heading for Column 2 in Table 10 to "…%reported in intervention versus control)". The way it reads now, it appears that the control group was much more likely to experience many adverse effects, particularly in Hall, 1998. It was only after a few minutes that I noticed footnote c indicating that the intervention group experienced more. So, I would keep the footnote but also have the order in the column heading consistent with the order reported in each row.	We agree and have made this change.
6	Page 23: It would be informative to have details of the disaggregated quality criteria scores for the included trials. As provided, I am not able to judge how trials scoring "fair" differed from those scoring "good". This would be best within the main body, but could be included in an appendix. Without these details, the transparency of the review is compromised, and the leap to GRADE in table 11 not clear.	We followed guidance in the EPC CER methods manual to report summary quality scores.
	Funnel plots are uninformative and unhelpful when there are small numbers of trials. In addition, the review has excluded any trials not published in peer reviewed journals, making the rationale for the funnel plots questionable. Thus, appendix D would be better removed.	We agree. The funnel plots were presented in the draft review for completeness but have been removed from the final review
	In forest plot figures, displaying the outcome number (eg figure 3, 1.2.1) is confusing to the reader. These should be removed from the plots.	This has been corrected.
	In forest plots with only 1 stratum of trials, please remove the bottom summary estimate – it merely duplicates the stratum summary estimate, complicates the plots and potentially confuses readers (eg figure 3 – remove "total" – it is same as "subtotal" estimate)	This has been corrected.
	In forest plots, it is helpful to order trials by the weight they contribute to the meta analysis – thus making in easier to see which trial contributes most to the summary estimate of effect, and also which are likely to be responsible for any heterogeneity.	We have made this change.
	Consistency of style and content among tables: table 9 page 34 includes a column marked "rating", with no further explanation. Presumably this reflects methodological quality? Similar tables preceding and following do not contain this column.	We have deleted this column.
	The evidence tables page 57 onwards are enormous and somewhat unwieldy. It is hard to see where one trial stops and another starts. Could these be reorganised so there is clearer delineation among trials? Certainly start each new trial at the top of a page, even separate table for each trial?	We have disaggregated the evidence tables. Each table starts on a new page.

45

APPENDIX C: EVIDENCE TABLES

Comparative Effectiveness of Smoking Cessation Treatments for Patients With Depression

Study ID: Brown, Kahler, Niaura, et al., 2001

Study Information	Interventions	Participant Characteristics	Results and Adverse Effects	Comments/ Quality Scoring
Geographical location: Providence, RI	**Intervention description:** Standard CBT for smoking cessation (ST) vs ST + CBT for depression (CBT-D)	**Inclusion criteria:** - Ages 18 to 70 - Smoked for at least 1 yr (10 cigarettes/ day) - History of MDD	**Follow-up rate:** 6 mo = 91% 12 mo = 92%	**General comments:** None
Recruitment: Advertisement; newspaper	ST = 93	**Exclusion criteria:** - Current depression	**Important baseline differences:** None	**Applicability cautions:** None
Setting: - Mixed - Academic	CBT = 86 Patients randomized to treatment condition according to gender, current depressive symptoms (BDI = 9), and level of nicotine	- Substance use - Current weekly psychotherapy - Use of other tobacco products - Intent to use pharmacological aid for	**Outcomes of interest** 1) Abstinence rate:	**Study-level quality assessment:** Good **Measure of smoking**
Veterans clinics: No	dependence	cessation	6 mo 12 mo	**adequate?** Yes
Study design: RCT	**Smoking cessation intervention:** Behavioral interventions	- Psychotropic therapy	ST 24.7 24.7 CBT 24.4 32.5	**Assessment of adverse effects adequate?** No
Number of participants enrolled: 179	Eight 2-hr group CBT sessions in 6 wk (2 sessions clustered around quit date) coled by two therapists (clinical psychologist postdoctoral fellows, interns in clinical psychologist, clinical	**Age:** Mean (SD): 45.1 (9.27)	**2) Medication adherence rate:** NR	
Duration of follow-up: End of treatment, 1, 6, 12 mo follow-up	psychologists) Key components of smoking cessation therapy included treatment rationale, self-monitoring, self-management, nicotine fading,	**Gender (n [%]):** Female 107 (59.8%)	**3) Differential effects by gender:** NA	
Methods of assessment Smoking status: 7 day point previous CO	relapse prevention, social support Drugs: None	**Race/ethnicity (n [%]):** White 174 (97.2%)	**4) Differential effects by depression status:** NA	
monitor **Depression status:** BDI	**Depression intervention:** Behavioral interventions Eight 2-hour group CBT sessions in 6 wk (2 sessions clustered	**Baseline depression assessment:** - SCID - BDI (cutoff ≥ 9)	**5) Differential effects by treatment sequencing:** NA **Report adverse effects?** No	
POMS	around quit date) coled by two therapists (clinical psych post-doctoral fellows, interns in clinical psych, clinical psychologists)	- Mean (SD) = 7.8 (6.31) **Smoking characteristics:** - FTND = 6.8 (1.93)		
	Comparator intervention(s) Smoking cessation intervention: Behavioral interventions	- Saliva cotinine = 383.7 ng/ml (170.59) **Comorbid conditions (n [%]):**		
	Eight 2-hour group smoking cessation only CBT sessions in 6 wk (2 sessions clustered around quit date) coled by two therapists (clinical psych postdoctoral fellows, interns in clinical psych, clinical psychologists)	- History of alcohol abuse 78 (43.6%) - History of drug abuse 60 (35.8%)		
	Drugs: None			
	Depression intervention: None			
	Mean contact time/proportion of sessions completed: Sessions attended out of 8 possible: - Control 5.8 of 8 = 72.5% - Intervention 5.9 of 8 = 73.7%			
	Treatment sequencing: Not done			

Comparative Effectiveness of Smoking Cessation Treatments for Patients With Depression

Study ID: Covey, Glassman, and Stetner, 1999

Study Information	Interventions	Participant Characteristics	Results and Adverse Effects	Comments/Quality Scoring
Geographical location: New York, NY	**Intervention description:** Study compared the added effectiveness of naltrexone to behavioral counseling (6 sessions) vs placebo treatment	**Inclusion criteria:** - Ages 18 to 65 - Smoked ≥ 20 cigarettes/day - Smoked before leaving house when awakened - Made at least 1 attempt to quit in the past	**Follow-up rate:** NR **Important baseline differences:** Age p < .004 Naltrexone 39.7 (8.0) yr Placebo 33.8 (8.2) yr	**General comments:** Differential dropout prior to quit date: -Naltrexone 10 of 40 (25%) - Placebo 2 of 40 (5%)
Recruitment: Advertisement	Behavioral counseling + Naltrexone (n = 40) vs behavioral counseling + placebo (n = 40)	**Exclusion criteria:** - Current or history of psychiatric disorder other than MDD; not clearly specified - Current major medical illness - Current MDD, substance abuse or psychotic disorder excluded	Naltrexone: 75% (30 of 40) patients started study, 25% dropped out prior to quit date Placebo: 95% (38 of 40) patients started study, 5% dropped out prior to quit date	Then differential dropout during study in the opposite direction: - Naltrexone 3 of 30 (10%) - Placebo 11 of 38 (29%); reason given was that the pill was not helpful
Setting: - Mental health clinic - Academic	**Smoking cessation intervention:** Behavioral interventions 6 individual sessions based on the American Lung Association smoking cessation program (modified) conducted by trained therapist	**Age:** Mean (SD): NR for whole sample Range 18 to 65	**Outcomes of interest** 3 mo NR for entire population 6 mo quit rate (n, %,OR, p) Naltrexone 30 (26.7) 1.9 ns Placebo 36 (15.2)	**Applicability cautions:** - Mean age < 40 - More than 60% female
Veterans clinics: No	Topics consisted of fading, target quit date and coping skills for cravings and withdrawal symptoms	**Gender (n [%]):** N (65) NR for entire sample Female Naltrexone 20.4 of 30 (68%) Placebo 22.8 of 38 (60%)	**1) Abstinence rate:** End of treatment (4 wk) Naltrexone 14 of 30 (46.7%) Placebo 10 of 38 (26.3%) OR 2.5, ns	**Study-level quality assessment:** Fair
Study design: RCT	Sessions held 3 and 5 days prior to quit date, then weekly x 1 mo	**Race/ethnicity (n [%]):** NR	**2) Medication adherence rate:** NR	**Comments:** - Poor description of exclusion criteria - Poor description of depression measure
Number of participants enrolled: 80 randomized 68 completed 52 data at 6 mo follow-up	**Drugs** Naltrexone, 25 mg/day 3 to 5 days prior to quit, increased to 50 mg/day on quit date, then increased to 75 mg/day if tolerated x 1 mo	**Baseline depression assessment:** - Schedule for Affective Disorders, Lifetime version - History of depression	**3) Differential effects by gender:** End of treatment (4 wk) OR Women (44) 3.5 Men (22) 1.4	- Unequal dropout rate prior to quit date - No ITT analysis with 25% dropout rate in one arm but only 5% in other
Duration of follow-up: 6 mo phone follow-up post end of 1 mo treatment	**Depression intervention:** None in addition to behavioral intervention		6 mo quit rate: Nal Pla OR p Women 27.8 7.4 4.6 .07	**Measure of smoking adequate?** Yes: cotinine
Methods of assessment **Smoking status:** - 7 day abstinence self-report	**Comparator intervention(s)** **Smoking cessation intervention:** Behavioral interventions Same 6 sessions as described above	**Smoking characteristics:** Mean (SD): Self-report usage: - Naltrexone 34.3 (11.9) cigarettes/day - Placebo 30.3 (10.1) cigarettes/day		**Assessment of adverse effects adequate?** Original study questionnaire
- Blood cotinine concentration < 15 ng/ml	**Drugs** Placebo, 25, 50, then 75 mg/day x 1 mo	**Cotinine level:** - Naltrexone: 262 (130) ng/ml - Placebo: 271 (110) ng/ml		
Depression status: Score for Schedule for Affective Disorders indicating depression– NR	**Depression intervention:** None, as above	**Comorbid conditions (n [%]):** History of major depression: - Total 37 of 68 (55%) - Naltrexone 12.6 of 30 (42%) - Placebo 20 of 38 (53%)		
	Mean contact time/proportion of sessions completed: 27 of 40 (67.5%) subjects in both arms completed the treatment; number of sessions attended NR **Treatment sequencing:** NA			

47

Comparative Effectiveness of Smoking Cessation Treatments
for Patients With Depression

Study ID: Covey, Glassman, and Stetner, 1999

Study Information	Interventions	Participant Characteristics	Results and Adverse Effects	Comments/ Quality Scoring

			4) Differential effects by depression status:
			4 wk OR only present or absent given
			Negative (32) 0.8
			Positive (36) 8.4
			
			6 mo quit rate:
			       Nal Pla OR
			Smokers 28.6 9.1 4.0 ns
			
			Within depressed (4 wk)
			Women (26) 4.4
			Men (10) 2.7
			
			6 mo quit rate:
			       Nal Pla OR p
			Women 22.2 0.0 3.4 .04
			
			5) Differential effects by treatment sequencing: NA
			
			Report adverse effects? Yes
			-11 naltrexone dropout
			- Minnesota Withdrawal Symptom Scale, 6 pt scale; side effects on original 3-point scale
			- List
			- Panic attack
			- Malaise
			- Sleeplessness
			- Lack of concentration
			- Nausea and vomiting
			- Disorientation
			- Tremors	

Study ID: Covey, Glassman, Stetner, et al., 2002

Study Information	Interventions	Participant Characteristics	Results and Adverse Effects	Comments/ Quality Scoring
Geographical location: New York, NY	**Intervention description:** 9-week double-blind trial of sertraline titrated to 200 mg daily (n = 68) vs placebo (n = 66) following 1 wk placebo run-in; both arms received behavioral intervention	**Inclusion criteria:** - ≥ 1 MDE that remitted ≥ 6 mo prior to study - Ages 18 to 70 - ≥ 20 cigarettes/day x ≥ 1 yr - ≥ Prior quit attempt - Decreased cigarettes by ≥ 50% on quit date	**Follow-up rate:** 100 of 134 (74.6%) at quit date; NR for intervention period	**General comments:** Table 2 gives AE rates but suspect scale
Recruitment: Advertisement	**Smoking cessation intervention:** Behavioral interventions		**Important baseline differences:** FTND lower for intervention group: 6.1 (2.4) vs 7.1 (2.4)	**Applicability cautions:** No concerns
Setting: NR	Weekly 45-minute individual behavioral session that included standard smoking cessation techniques (orientation to health risk, benefits of cessation, coping skills for withdrawal symptoms and avoiding relapse)	**Exclusion criteria:** - Serious medical illness - Psychotropic medication - MDD - Alcohol or drug dependence - PTSD, panic disorder, bulimia, anorexia nervosa within past 6 mo - Other lifetime major Axis I disorders - Pregnancy	**Outcomes of interest** **1) Abstinence rate:** Post-quit day (randomization) Wk 6 (10): 19 of 66 (28.8%) placebo vs 23 of 68 (33.8%) intervention Wk 30 (34): 11 of 66 (16.7%) placebo vs 8 of 68 (11.8%) When analysis was limited to the 100 subjects enrolled until quit date, there were no statistically significant differences in abstinence rates	**Study-level quality assessment:** Good **Measure of smoking adequate?** Yes **Assessment of adverse effects adequate?** No
Veterans clinics: No	**Drugs** Sertraline 50 mg daily wk 1 100 mg daily wk 2 150 mg daily wk 3 200 mg daily wk 4-9 9 day medication taper			
Study design: RCT				
Number of participants enrolled: 66 placebo 68 sertraline	**Depression intervention:** Behavioral interventions	**Age:** Mean (SD): 44.5 (10.7)	**2) Medication adherence rate:** NR	
	Smoking cessation intervention augmented with a supportive approach to manage negative affect	**Gender (n [%]):** Female 85 (63.4%)	**3) Differential effects by gender:** NR	
Duration of follow-up: 34 week post-randomization		**Race/ethnicity (n [%]):** White 117 (87.3%)	**4) Differential effects by depression status:** No interaction effect for treatment by single vs recurrent depression or baseline depression status	
Methods of assessment	**Comparator intervention(s)** **Smoking cessation intervention:** Behavioral interventions Same as intervention	**Baseline depression assessment:** BDI-21 8.0 (7.7) CES-D 14.9 (10.8) HDRS 4.8 (4.4)		
Smoking status: Self-report for 7 days and serum cotinine < 25 ng/ml	Drugs: Placebo	**Smoking characteristics:** * - Yr smoking: 25.4 (10.5), 26.6 (10.8) - Cigarettes/day: 29.6 (11.5), 26.9 (9.0) - FTND: 7.1 (2.4), 6.1 (2.4) * = Placebo, intervention	**5) Differential effects by treatment sequencing:** NA	
Depression status: 6 point unvalidated scale	**Depression intervention:** Behavioral intervention Same as intervention	**Comorbid conditions:** NR	**Report adverse effects?** Yes -Dizziness, agitation, spaciness, diarrhea	
	Mean contact time/proportion of sessions completed: 9 visits during 12 wk intervention, each lasting about 45 min		-7 placebo, 4 intervention dropped out by wk 4 due to AE	
	Treatment sequencing: NA			

Study ID: Duffy, Ronis, Valenstein, et al, 2006

Study Information	Interventions	Participant Characteristics	Results and Adverse Effects	Comments/ Quality Scoring
Geographical location: - University of Michigan, VAMC, Ann Arbor, MI - VAMC, Dallas, TX - VAMC, Gainesville, FL **Recruitment:** Clinic waiting room at study sites **Setting:** - Primary care - Academic and nonacademic, mixed **Veterans clinics:** Yes **Study design:** RCT **Number of participants enrolled:** 184 enrolled 91 usual care 93 intervention **Duration of follow-up:** 6 mo from end of intervention **Methods of assessment** **Smoking status:** - Self-report - Abstinent at least 1 mo to be "quitter," reported at 6 mo follow-up - No biochemical measure **Depression status:** NR	**Intervention description:** Combined smoking, depression, alcohol abuse telephone counseling (n = 93) vs enhanced usual care of brief counseling and referral to appropriate services for substance use/abuse and/or depression (n = 91) All participants were nonterminal head and neck cancer patients **Smoking cessation intervention:** Behavioral interventions 45 min baseline assessment and brief counseling with RN using semistructured instruments CBT, 9-11 sessions, planned telephone counseling and workbook Therapist was RN trained specifically for intervention Topics included tobacco tactics, drinking decisions, and mood management using goal setting, self-monitoring, analyzing behavioral antecedents, coping, and social skills training Drugs - Offered as needed - Nicotine replacement and/or bupropion **Depression intervention:** Behavioral interventions: None additional Drugs Offered antidepressants on individual basis (bupropion, paroxetine, fluoxetine, sertraline) **Comparator intervention(s)** **Smoking cessation intervention:** Behavioral interventions 45 min baseline assessment and brief counseling with RN using semistructured instruments Referred as needed to smoking cessation, alcohol treatment, or mental health evaluation according to insurance and ability to pay (options and time spent standardized) Handout listing all services available in area (e.g., Alcoholics Anonymous) Drugs Not specified as prescribed on individual basis **Depression intervention:** Behavioral interventions See above, dependent on individual referral Drugs: None specified **Mean contact time/proportion of sessions completed:** 77 of 93 (82.8%) completed all aspects of intervention **Treatment sequencing:** NA	**Inclusion criteria:** - Diagnosis head and neck cancer - Comorbid smoking, depression, or problem drinking - Older than age 18 - HDRS >20 or severe drinking **Exclusion criteria:** - Pregnant - Non-English - Terminal illness - Unstable psychiatric illness **Age:** 57 (9.9) **Gender (n [%]) :** Male 155 (84%) **Race/ethnicity (n [%]):** White 166, (90%) Other 18 (10%) **Baseline depression assessment:** Geriatric Depression Scale-short form; score > 4 at baseline and follow-up (69% of sample depressed) **Smoking characteristics:** Self report; 74% of sample **Comorbid conditions (n [%]):** - Depression 127 (69%) - Alcohol 52 (28%)	**Follow-up rate:** 84% at 6 mo for total population **Important baseline differences:** None **Outcomes of interest** - Quit rate at 6 mo for all smokers (n = 136) - Intervention, 35 of 74 (47%) - Usual care, 19 of 62 (31%) 1) **Abstinence rate:** At 6 mo for those depressed at baseline (n = 64): Intervention 51% (18 of 35) Usual care 17% (5 of 29) 2) **Medication adherence rate:** NR 3) **Differential effects by gender:** NR 4) **Differential effects by depression status:** NR 5) **Differential effects by treatment sequencing:** Not done **Report adverse effects?** No List	**General comments:** This study tried to treat smoking, alcohol abuse, and depression concomitantly in a group of head and neck cancer survivors Only 64 participants had depression and also smoked at baseline Depression was mild to moderate and excluded those with HDRS > 20 Used Geriatric Depression Scale-short form > 4 to define depressed **Applicability cautions:** Good; 52% vets, correct age, male; all head and neck cancer patients **Study-level quality assessment:** Good **Measure of smoking adequate?** No; no biochemical validation of self-report status; self-report alone may underestimate current smokers **Assessment of adverse effects adequate?** No

Comparative Effectiveness of Smoking Cessation Treatments for Patients With Depression

Evidence-basedSynthesisProgram

Study ID: Evins, Culhane, Alpert, et al., 2008

Study Information	Interventions	Participant Characteristics	Results and Adverse Effects	Comments/ Quality Scoring
Geographical location: Boston, MA	**Intervention description:** Intervention = 97 Comparator = 102	**Inclusion criteria:** - Ages 18 to 70 - Smoked > 10 cigarettes/day for more than 2 yr - Lifetime diagnosis of UDD (so current and history of depression) - History of depression or current depression	**Follow-up rate:** 99 of 199 = 49.7%	**General comments:** None
Recruitment: - Advertisement - Referral	Blocked randomization on level of nicotine dependence, failed history of treatment with NRT and/or CBT, current or past UDD		**Important baseline differences:** More men and fewer depression episodes in placebo arm	**Applicability cautions:** Very high dropout rate
Setting: - Mixed - Academic	13 sessions of group CBT + 8 wk NRT + 12 wk bupropion SR vs 13 sessions of group CBT + 8 wk NRT + placebo		**Outcomes of interest**	**Study-level quality assessment:** Good
Veterans clinics: No	**Smoking cessation intervention:** Behavioral interventions	**Exclusion criteria:** - Substance use disorder - Other psychiatric disorders	1) **Abstinence rate:** At 13 wk post-baseline: 36% bupropion and 31% placebo using intent to treat analyses	**Measure of smoking adequate?** Yes
Study design: RCT	13 wk of group CBT with groups up to 6 patients plus weekly visit with study psychiatrist (session 1 treatment rationale; session 2, cognitive behavioral suggestions for using NRT; sessions 3 to 13, cognitive behavioral strategies of maintenance of abstinence)	- Current use of nicotine-containing products, psychotropic medications, or behavioral smoking cessation treatment	2) **Medication adherence rate:** NR	**Assessment of adverse effects adequate?** NA
Number of participants enrolled: 199		**Age:** Mean (SD): 43 (11)	3) **Differential effects by gender:** Not done	
Duration of follow-up: 13 wk	These CBT sessions did not address depression	**Gender (n [%]):** Female 97 (49%)	4) **Differential effects by depression status:** Yes - Current UDD:	
	Depression intervention: None	**Race/ethnicity (n [%]):** NA	33% (15 of 45) bupropion vs 31% (14 of 45) in placebo were abstinent	
Methods of assessment Smoking status: 7 day self-report CO validated ≤ ppm	**Comparator intervention(s) Smoking cessation intervention:** Behavioral interventions	**Baseline depression assessment:** HAM-D-6	- History of UDD: 39% (20 of 52) bupropion vs 32% (18 of 57) in placebo were abstinent	
Depression status: HAM-D-6:	Same as above: 13 wk of group CBT with groups up to 6 patients plus weekly visit with study psychiatrist These CBT sessions did not address depression	**Smoking characteristics:** - 7 day point prevalence - FNTD	5) **Differential effects by treatment sequencing:** Not done	
HAM-D-6: > 4 high ≤ 4 low	**Drugs** - Bupropion 12 wk (150 mg/day for 3 days and then 150 mg BID) - NRT 8 wk (21 mg patches for wk 2 to 6; 14 mg patches wk 7 and 8; 7 mg patches wk 9 and 10) **Depression intervention:** None	**Comorbid conditions (n [%]):** Lifetime anxiety 79 (40%)	**Report adverse effects?** No	
	Drugs - NRT 8 wk (21 mg patches for wk 2 to 6; 14 mg patches wk 7 and 8; 7 mg patches wk 9 and 10) - Placebo 12 wk (same schedule as bupropion) **Depression intervention:** None			
	Mean contact time/proportion of sessions completed: NR, but 50% dropped out **Treatment sequencing:** NA			

Study ID: Hall, Munoz, and Reus, 1994

Study Information	Interventions	Participant Characteristics	Results and Adverse Effects	Comments/ Quality Scoring
Geographical location: San Francisco, CA	**Intervention description:** 5 sessions of small group smoking cessation treatment + 5 sessions of CBT mood management + nicotine gum vs 5 sessions of small group smoking cessation treatment + nicotine gum	**Inclusion criteria:** - 10+ cigarettes per day - Ages 18 to 65	**Follow-up rate:** NR; subjects with missing data were coded as smoking	**General comments:** None
Recruitment: - Patients responding to "announcements" - Referred by physician or friend	MDD history negative: Control n = 53 CBT n = 50 MDD history positive: Control n = 17 CBT n = 29	**Exclusion criteria:** - Heart disease - Angina, vasospastic disease - Current or past peptic ulcer - Temporomandibular joint disease - Hypertension - Life-threatening illness - Alcohol or drug problems in past 6 mo - Current treatment for psychiatric problems - History of psychiatric hospitalization in past yr - Pregnant or nursing - Current MDD screened out	**Important baseline differences:** NR	**Applicability cautions:** - Current MDD or other psychiatric treatment excluded - Volunteer reactive sample
Setting: - Research clinic - Academic medical center	**Smoking cessation intervention:** Behavioral interventions Ten 2-hr sessions over 8 wk (2 x for first 2 wk) First 5 sessions were "standard" smoking treatment: information on smoking, gum use, quit plan Intervention was delivered by 1 MD from preventive medicine specialty and 1 PhD psychologist		**Outcomes of interest** **1) Abstinence rate:** Wk 12 rates (from baseline)	**Study-level quality assessment:** Fair to poor
Veterans clinics: No	Drugs - NRT, 2 mg gum as needed for 8 wk - Taper at 9-12 wk - Mo 4-6 carry "shelf" gum for high-risk situations	**Age:** Mean (SD): 40.6 (9.2)	MDD history negative: Control 26 of 53 (49%) CBT 23 of 50 (46%)	**Comments:** - Randomization and allocation NR - Baseline characteristics by intervention NR - Follow-up rates NR - Adherence NR - Dropout NR
Study design: RCT	**Depression intervention:** Behavioral interventions 5 sessions of CBT focused on mood management: - Monitoring of thoughts, daily activities, interpersonal contacts and mood	**Gender (n [%]):** Men 71 (48%) Women 78 (52%)	MDD history positive: Control 8 of 17 (47%) CBT 20 of 29 (69%)	
Number of participants enrolled: 149	- Focus on increasing thoughts and activities related to healthy mood and to not smoking - Increasing pleasant activities - Increasing pleasant social contacts - Relation training - Identifying and modifying maladaptive thoughts - Setting realist life goals (manual available)	**Race/ethnicity (n [%]):** White 131 (88%)	Wk 52	**Measure of smoking adequate?** Yes
Duration of follow-up: 8, 12, 26, 52 wk	**Comparator intervention(s)** **Smoking cessation intervention:** Behavioral interventions 5 sessions, 8 wk	**Baseline depression assessment:** - DIS used to assess history of MDD, n = 46 (31%) history positive	MDD history negative: Control 13 of 53 (25%) CBT 8 of 50 (16%)	**Assessment of adverse effects adequate?** NR
Methods of assessment **Smoking status:** - Biologically verified self-report of 7-day abstinence from cigarettes: expired CO ≤10 ppm - At 52 wk CO measured and urinary cotinine ≤ 60 ng/ml	Small group; only support; leader did not condone any specific suggestions or offered any	- BDI: History positive n = 6.39 (5.9) History negative n = 4.58 (4.6)	MDD history positive: Control 4 of 17 (24%) CBT 10 of 29 (34%)	
Depression status: - BDI-II NR at follow-up - Profile of mood states reported	Drugs: Gum as above **Depression intervention:** None **Mean contact time/proportion of sessions completed:** NR **Treatment sequencing:** NA	**Smoking characteristics:** 24.9 (10.9) cigarettes/day 26.7 (13.9) CO level FTND tolerance scale 6.4 (1.9) Regular smoking yr 22.1 (9.5) **Comorbid conditions:** NR	**2) Medication adherence rate:** NR	
			3) Differential effects by gender: NR	
			4) Differential effects by depression status: See above for unadjusted rates; the diagnosis x treatment group interaction was significant Among only those with MDD history positive, 10 of 29 (34%) vs 3 of 17 (18%) at 1 yr	
			5) Differential effects by treatment sequencing: NA **Report adverse effects?** No	

Study ID: Hall, Munoz, Reus, et al., 1996

Study Information	Interventions	Participant Characteristics	Results and Adverse Effects	Comments/ Quality Scoring
Geographical location: San Francisco, CA	**Intervention description:** 2 (behavioral treatments) x 2 (gum vs placebo) factorial design; stratified by MDD history and cigarettes smoked	**Inclusion criteria:** - 10+ cigarettes per day - Ages 18 to 65	**Follow-up rate:** NR; subjects with missing data were coded as smoking	**General comments:** **Caution:** 2 x 2 factorial but data presented as if a 4-arm study, so each subject is double counted
Recruitment: Media, fliers, word of mouth	Both behavioral arms 10-session group over 8 wk; quit date set for third group session; groups 5-12 patients	**Exclusion criteria:** - Heart disease - Ulcers	**Important baseline differences:** NR	
Setting: - Research clinic - Academic medical center	(Cell sizes in 2 x 2 NR; n's below collapse across 1 treatment condition)	- Oral thrush - Current alcohol or drug problems - Hypertension	**Outcomes of interest** No effect for treatment gum dose, MDD history, or interaction	**Applicability cautions:** - Current MDD or other psychiatric treatment excluded - Volunteer reactive sample - Participants had to pay $75 deposit
Veterans clinics: No	MDD history negative: Health education (control) n = 74 CBT n = 83	- Pregnancy - Current mental health treatment - Use of psychoactive drugs	**1) Abstinence rate:** Wk 12 rates (from baseline)	
Study design: RCT	Placebo gum n = 82 Active gum n = 75	- Physician letter indicating that patient is healthy	MDD history negative: Control: 26 of 74 (35%) CBT: 29 of 83 (35%)	**Study-level quality assessment:** Fair
Number of participants enrolled: 207, but 201 analyzed; 6 excluded because of protocol violations (e.g., use of nicotine patch)	MDD history positive: Control n = 23 CBT n = 21	- Current MDD excluded **Age:** Mean (SD): 39.7 (NR) Range: 22 to 65	Placebo gum: 28 of 82 (34%) Active gum: 27 of 75 (36%) MDD history positive: Control: 8 of 23 (35%)	**Comments:** - Randomization and allocation NR - Baseline characteristics by treatment group NR
	Placebo gum n = 21 Active gum n = 23	**Gender (n [%]):** Women 105 (52%) Men 96 (48%)	CBT: 10 of 21 (48%) Placebo gum: 11 of 21 (52%) Active gum: 7 of 23 (30%)	- Follow-up rates NR - Adherence NR - Dropout NR
Duration of follow-up: - 8 wk (treatment termination)	**Smoking cessation intervention:** Behavioral interventions Ten 2-hr sessions based on Hall 1994	**Race/ethnicity (n [%]):** White 185 (92%)	Wk 52 MDD history negative: Control: 17 of 74 (23%)	**Measure of smoking adequate?** Yes
- 12 wk post–treatment termination + 26 and 52 wk post–treatment termination	"Mood management" CBT focused as described in Hall 1994; "standard" smoking treatment: information on smoking, gum use, quit plan	**Baseline depression assessment:** - DIS used to assess history of MDD; 22% of 201 history positive - BDI 6.71 (5.43)	CBT: 23 of 83 (28%) Placebo gum: 21 of 82 (26%) Active gum: 19 of 75 (25%)	**Assessment of adverse effects adequate?** NR
Methods of assessment **Smoking status:** - Biologically verified self-report of 7-day abstinence from cigarettes: expired CO ≤10 ppm - At 52 wk CO measured and urinary cotinine ≤60 ng/ml	Intervention was delivered by weekly supervision from PhD psychologist including review of audiotapes **Drugs** - NRT: 2 mg gum at session 3 (quit date) for 8 wk - Chew at least 1 piece per hr for at least 12 hr/day during first 3 wk - Use prn wk 4-8 - Taper at 9-12 weeks - Mo 4-6 carry "shelf" gum for high-risk situations - By 6 mo abstinent from all NRT	**Smoking characteristics:** - 23.8 (9.8) cigarettes/day - 27.2 (11.81) CO level - Regular smoking yr 21 (NR) **Comorbid conditions:** NR	MDD history positive: Control: 5 of 23 (22%) CBT: 7 of 21 (33%) Placebo gum: 7 of 21 (33%) Active gum: 5 of 23 (22%) **2) Medication adherence rate:** NR **3) Differential effects by gender:** NR **4) Differential effects by depression status:** See above for unadjusted rates; the diagnosis x treatment group interaction was not significant **5) Differential effects by treatment sequencing:** NA **Report adverse effects?** No	
Depression status: - BDI-II not related to MDD history - Profile of mood states higher at wk 2 post-quit with increase for MDD history positive				

Study ID: Hall, Munoz, Reus, et al., 1996

Study Information	Interventions	Participant Characteristics	Results and Adverse Effects	Comments/ Quality Scoring
	Depression intervention: Behavioral interventions 5 of CBT focused on mood management: - Monitoring of thoughts, daily activities, interpersonal contacts and mood - Focus on increasing thoughts and activities related to healthy mood and to not smoking - Increasing pleasant activities - Increasing pleasant social contacts - Relation training - Identifying and modifying maladaptive thoughts - Setting realistic life goals (manual available) **Comparator intervention(s)** **Smoking cessation intervention:** Behavioral interventions Group health education "Standard" smoking treatment: information on smoking, gum use, quit plan developed and modified each week Group leader provided health information and facilitated group discussion **Drugs** As above **Depression intervention:** None **Mean contact time/proportion of sessions completed:** NR **Treatment sequencing:** NA			

Comparative Effectiveness of Smoking Cessation Treatments for Patients With Depression

Study ID: Hall, Reus, Munoz, et al., 1998

Study Information	Interventions	Participant Characteristics	Results and Adverse Effects	Comments/ Quality Scoring
Geographical location: San Francisco, CA **Recruitment:** - Public service announcements - Newspaper ads **Setting:** - Research clinic - Academic medical center **Veterans clinics:** No **Study design:** RCT **Number of participants enrolled:** 199 **Duration of follow-up:** - 8 wk (treatment termination) - 12 weeks post-treatment termination plus 26 and 52 wk post-treatment termination **Methods of assessment** **Smoking status:** - Biologically verified self-report of 7-day abstinence from cigarettes: expired CO $\leq$10 ppm - Urinary cotinine $\leq$341 nmol/l **Depression status:** - BDI - Profile of mood states reported for only 8 days after quit	**Intervention description:** 2 (CBT vs health education) x 2 (nortriptyline vs placebo) Drug/CBT (n = 51) MDD history positive n = 17 (33.3%) Drug/health education (n = 48) MDD history positive n = 15 (31.3%) Placebo/CBT (n = 52) MDD history positive n = 17 (32.7%) Placebo/health education (n = 48) MDD history positive n = 16 (33.3) **Smoking cessation intervention:** Behavioral interventions Group "mood management" CBT as described in Hall 1994 Ten 2-hr group sessions over 8 wk Group size 5-11 patients CBT focused on mood management skills to manage dysphoria and maintain nonsmoking and included methods to increase the frequency of pleasant activities and decrease relapse-related thoughts and techniques for increasing positive social contacts, decreasing negative contacts, and improving relationships. Intervention delivered by 3 PhD psychologists **Drugs** Double blind; MD visits wk 1, 2, 3 Nortriptyline hydrochloride at therapeutic dose for depression; 25 mg/day for 3 days; increased to 50 mg/day for 4 days Serum assessed at wk 2 Dose increased to 75 mg/day if therapeutic level not attained; increased to 100 mg/day if necessary at wk 6 Modal dose 100 mg/day; maintenance to wk 12 Taper during wk 13 (whenever active drug was titrated; someone in placebo was titrated) **Depression intervention:** Behavioral interventions 5 sessions of CBT (smoking/mood management) as above	**Inclusion criteria:** - 10+ cigarettes per day - Ages 21 to 65 **Exclusion criteria:** - Heart disease or ECG abnormalities - "Other reasons" - Current mental health treatment - Use of psychoactive drugs - Current MDD - Alcohol or other non-nicotine drug use **Age:** Mean (SD): Drug + CBT 41.7 (9.4) Drug + health education: 40.7 (9.6) Placebo + CBT: 40.0 (9.9) Placebo + health education: 39.4 (9.7) **Gender (n [%]):** Women n = 110 (55%) Men n = 89 (45%) **Race/ethnicity (n [%]):** White 173 (89%) **Baseline depression assessment:** DIS used to assess history of MDD: MDD history positive n = 65 (32.7) BDI: MDD history positive n = 7.2 (5.6) MDD history negative n = 5.5 (2.2) **Smoking characteristics:** Range of mean (SD) for the 4 groups: - FTND 5.4 (2.2) to 5.2 (2.2) - Yr smoking 21.7 (10.0) to 23.0 (10.7) - Daily cigarettes 21.1 (7.6) to 24.9 (12.1) **Comorbid conditions:** NR	**Follow-up rate:** N = 47 (24%) dropped out of treatment No difference in psychological intervention or history of MDD in dropout rates but dropout higher in placebo drug (30%) vs active drug (17%) (or = 2.01; 1.05-4.06) **Important baseline differences:** None **Outcomes of interest** **1) Abstinence rate:** ITT analyses abstracted here: Wk 12 rates (from baseline) MDD history negative: Drug + CBT 56%, 19 of 34 Drug + health education 61%, 20 of 33 Placebo + CBT 20%,7 of 35 Placebo + health education 31%, 10 of 32 MDD history positive: Drug + CBT 47%, 8 of 17 Drug + health education 47%, 7 of 15 Placebo + CBT 41%,7 of 17 Placebo + health education 19%,3 of 16 Wk 64 MDD history negative: Drug + CBT 35%, 12 of 34 Drug + health education 36%, 12 of 33 Placebo + CBT 20%, 7 of 35 Placebo + health education 22%, 7 of 32 MDD history positive: Drug + CBT 24%, 4 of 17 Drug + health education 20%, 3 to 15 Placebo + CBT 29%, 5 of 17 Placebo + health education 13%, 2 of 16	**General comments:** Randomization stratified by depression status **Applicability cautions:** - Current MDD or other psychiatric treatment excluded - Volunteer reactive sample **Study-level quality assessment:** Good Comments: Adherence rate to behavioral treatment NR **Measure of smoking adequate?** Yes **Assessment of adverse effects adequate?** Yes

Study ID: Hall, Reus, Munoz, et al., 1998

Study Information	Interventions	Participant Characteristics	Results and Adverse Effects	Comments/ Quality Scoring
	Comparator intervention(s) **Smoking cessation intervention:** Behavioral interventions Group health education Group leader provided health information and facilitated group discussion Development of quit plan; modified quit plan each week but only five 90-min sessions (5-11 patients per group) over 8 wk. Methods included paper-and-pencil exercises, informational handouts, brief didactic presentations, homework assignments, and smoking monitoring Drugs: As above **Depression intervention:** Behavioral interventions: Drug as above **Mean contact time/proportion of sessions completed:** NR **Treatment sequencing:** NA		**2) Medication adherence rate:** Capsules did not differ by condition or drug (active vs placebo) **3) Differential effects by gender:** Gender by MDD history interaction significant; MDD history positive women had poorer abstinence rates than MDD history negative (or =2.05; 1.32-3.23) but not for MDD history positive men (p = 0.20) Women: Wk 12 MDD history positive 38% MDD history negative 53% Wk 64 MDD history positive 20% MDD history negative 37% Men: Wk 12 MDD history positive 61% MDD history negative 52% Wk 64 MDD history positive 37% MDD history negative 31% **4) Differential effects by depression status:** See above for unadjusted rates for main effect for drug; 24% vs 12% placebo achieved continuous abstinence The diagnosis (i.e., MDD history) by psychological treatment by drug interaction was not significant Behavioral treatment condition by MDD history was significant	

Study ID: Hall, Reus, Munoz, et al., 1998

Study Information	Interventions	Participant Characteristics	Results and Adverse Effects	Comments/ Quality Scoring
			MDD history positive assigned to CBT did as well as MDD history negative	
			MDD history positive assigned to control were less likely to be abstinent than those assigned to CBT	
			Drug by diagnosis was not significant	
			The diagnosis x treatment group interaction was not significant	
			5) Differential effects by treatment sequencing: NA **Report adverse effects?** - Measured by checklist - Dry mouth 78% drug vs 33% or 7.0; 95% CI 3.73 to 13.17 - Lightheaded 49% vs 22% or 2.42 1.85-6.35 - Shaky hands 23% vs 11% or 2.42; 1.11-5.29 - Blurry vision 16% vs 6% 3.00; 1.12-7.99	

Comparative Effectiveness of Smoking Cessation Treatments for Patients With Depression

Study ID: Hall, Tsoh, Prochaska, et al., 2006

Study Information	Interventions	Participant Characteristics	Results and Adverse Effects	Comments/Quality Scoring
Geographical location: San Francisco, CA	**Intervention description:** Brief contact and referral control (n = 159) vs staged-care intervention (n = 163)	**Inclusion criteria:** - Diagnosis of current depression based on PRIME MD	**Follow-up rate:** 3 mo: Control (n = 129; 81%) Intervention (n = 138; 85%)	**General comments:** None
Recruitment: - Provider referral - Invitation letters to clinic patients - Flyers in clinics - Paid $150	**Smoking cessation intervention:** Behavioral interventions Computerized motivational feedback based on the stages of change model (15 min session given at baseline, 3, 6, and 12 mo) Patients at contemplation stage were also offered counseling	- Smoked 1+ cigarettes/day in week prior to enrollment - Enrollment as a patient in one of four participating sites **Exclusion criteria:** - Under age 18	6 mo: Control (n = 120; 75%) Intervention (n = 125; 77%) 12 mo: Control (n = 112; 70%) Intervention (n = 113; 69%)	**Applicability cautions:** - Patients recruited from large HMO - Patients did not need to have intention to quit to enroll
Setting: - Mental health outpatient clinics - Academic and nonacademic	Cessation treatment program of CBT; six 30 min sessions of individual treatments over 8 wk offered by one of two therapists (MA-level psychologist or PhD psychologist)	- Non-English speaking - History of bipolar - Contraindicated to use of pharmacological treatments - Dementia or other disorders interfering with comprehension of materials	18 mo: Control (n = 110; 69%) Intervention (n = 122; 75%) **Important baseline differences:** Control had higher % of lifetime nicotine dependence: 74.7% vs 64.2% (not correlated with outcomes)	**Study-level quality assessment:** Good **Measure of smoking adequate?** Yes **Assessment of adverse effects adequate?** NR
Veterans clinics: No **Study design:** RCT	CBT consisted of quit plan that was iteratively revised, quite date, self-tests about reasons for smoking, information about risks/ benefits of quitting, information on nutrition and exercise, mood monitoring, discussion of ways to increase pleasant moods and decrease negative ones, use of behavioral skills to reduce relapse risk, and relation and social support skills.	**Age:** Mean (SD): Control (n = 159) 42.2 (12.8) Staged care (n = 163) 41.5 (12.4) Median: NR Range: NR	**Outcomes of interest** **1) Abstinence rate** Rates based on ITT analyses (missing = smoker)	
Number of participants enrolled: 322 **Duration of follow-up:** 18 mo	**Drugs** - NRT - If smoked 10+ cigarettes got 21 mg patch for 6 wk, 14 mg wk 7-8; 7 mg wk 9-10 - If failed NRT, could request bupropion (dose NR)	**Gender (n [%]):** Male 98 (30.4%) Female 224 (69.6%)	Intervention: 3 mo: 22 of 163 (13.5%) 6 mo: 23 of 163 (14.11%) 12 mo: 23 of 163 (14.11%) 18 mo: 30 of 163 (18.4%)	
Methods of assessment **Smoking status:** - Biologically verified self-report of 7-day abstinence from cigarettes: expired $CO \leq 10$ ppm - Interviewers blind to treatment group	**Depression intervention:** None **Comparator intervention(s)** **Smoking cessation intervention:** Behavioral interventions Brief contact; list of referrals to smoking cessation programs and stop smoking guide	**Race/ethnicity (n [%]):** White 220 (68.3%) **Baseline depression assessment:** PRIME-MD + to be enrolled **BDI-II:** Control 21.4 (10.9) Staged care 20.6 (11.7)	Control: 3 mo: 15 of 159 (9.43%) 6 mo: 25 of 159 (15.73%) 12 mo: 15 of 159 (9.43%) 18 mo: 21 of 159 (13.21%) Gee model:	
Depression status: BDI-II	**Drugs:** None **Depression intervention:** None **Mean contact time/proportion of sessions completed:** NR **Treatment sequencing:** See above	**DIS** **DSM-IV + MDD:** Control 155 (97.5) Staged care 152 (93.3) Current MDD: Control 133 (83.7) Staged care 135 (82.8) Recurrent MDD: Control 89 (57.4) Staged care 79 (52.0)	Main effect for treatment at 12 and 18 mo (completed only on responders) OR = 4.459 (95%) CI = 1.04 to 19.93 P = 0.0441 **2) Medication adherence rate:** NR	

Study ID: Hall, Tsoh, Prochaska, et al., 2006

Study Information	Interventions	Participant Characteristics	Results and Adverse Effects	Comments/ Quality Scoring
		Smoking characteristics: FTND: Control 4.2 (2.6) Staged care 3.8 (2.4) Number of cigarettes/day: Control 15.3 (10.3) Staged care 15.8 (10.0) CO at baseline: Control 15.2 (10.2) Staged care 15.5 (9.9) **Comorbid conditions:** NR	**3) Differential effects by gender:** NR **4) Differential effects by depression status:** - BDI-II not related to outcomes - Analyses conducted in only MDD (n = 307) with same pattern of results; results not shown **5) Differential effects by treatment sequencing:** NA **Report adverse effects?** No	

Comparative Effectiveness of Smoking Cessation Treatments for Patients With Depression

Study ID: Hayford, Patten, Rummans, et al., 1999

Study Information	Interventions	Participant Characteristics	Results and Adverse Effects	Comments/Quality Scoring
Geographical location: Three U.S. sites: Palo Alto, CA Rochester, MN Morgantown, WV	**Intervention description:** 100 mg bupropion + behavioral intervention (n = 153) vs 150 mg + behavioral intervention (n = 153) vs 300 mg + behavioral intervention n = 156) vs placebo (n = 153)	**Inclusion criteria:** - Age ≥ 18 - Smoked ≥ 15 cigarettes/day for past yr - Motivated to stop smoking - Good general health	**Follow-up rate:** 396 of 615 (64%) completed 12 mo follow-up	**General comments:** Effect of dose was dependent on diagnosis group
Recruitment: Advertisement	**Smoking cessation intervention:** Behavioral interventions - Set target quit date after 1 wk of medication - Personalized message to stop smoking - Self-help materials based on NCI program - Brief in-person individual counseling (10-15 min) by study assistant at weekly visits x 7 wk, then at 8, 12, 26, and 52 wk - Telephoned 3 days after target quit date and at 4, 5, 7, 8, 9, 10, and 11 mo	**Exclusion criteria:** - History of head trauma, predisposition to seizures, anorexia nervosa, or bulimia - Current depression - Pregnancy - History of alcohol or substance abuse within past yr - Personal or family history of seizure disorder - Psychotropic medication use or NRT - Previous use of bupropion - Use of other tobacco products	Completion varied by bupropion group: 57% (100 mg), 65% (150 mg), 64% (300 mg), 71% (placebo), p = 0.01	**Applicability cautions:** - Mean age < 45 - 96% white - 55% female
Setting: - Mental health, primary care, mixed - Academic and nonacademic			**Important baseline differences:** None between randomized groups; there were important differences between those with and without history of MDD or alcohol dependence (age, gender); however, mean changes in BDI scores did not significantly differ from zero for any group	**Study-level quality assessment:** Good
Veterans clinics: No	**Drugs** - Bupropion SR 50 mg BID - Bupropion SR 150 mg am + placebo pm - Bupropion SR 150 mg daily x 3 days, then 150 mg BID - All drugs given for 7 wk			**Comments:** - Allocation concealment not specified - Differential follow-up rate, if dropout, assumed to be smoking and would bias against intervention - Funded by Glaxo Wellcome and included industry investigator(s)
Study design: RCT, 4 arms	**Depression intervention:** None	**Age:** Mean (SD): 42 to 43 Median: NR Range: NR	**Outcomes of interest** **1) Abstinence rate:** 3 and 12 mo rates (% of randomized)	
Number of participants enrolled: 742 volunteers 615 eligible and randomized	**Comparator intervention(s)** **Smoking cessation intervention:** Behavioral interventions Same as intervention groups	**Gender (n [%]):** Female 336 (54.6%)	Placebo: 14.4%;12.4% 100 mg: 24.2%; 19.6% 150 mg: 26.1%; 22.9% 300 mg: 29.5%; 23.1%	**Measure of smoking adequate?** Yes
Duration of follow-up: 3 mo and 12 mo from baseline		**Race/ethnicity (n [%]):** White 591(96%)	p = 0.01 at 3 mo; p = 0.06 at 12 mo for all 4 groups 150 mg and 300 mg doses statistically significant compared to placebo at all time points	**Assessment of adverse effects adequate?** Fair; measured depressive symptoms and weight change but little detail on other AE measures
Methods of assessment	**Drugs** Placebo BID for 7 wk, n = 153	**Baseline depression assessment:** BDI-21, score range 0-63		
Smoking status: Self-reported abstinence for 7 days verified by CO level ≤10 ppm	**Depression intervention:** None	Mean (SD) ranges from 4.1 (4.2) to 4.7 (5.0)	12 mo rates for participants with history of MDD	
Depression status: BDI-21 item	**Mean contact time/proportion of sessions completed:** 467 of 615 (75%) completed 7 wk intervention	SCID for lifetime MDD, total n = 114	Placebo: 2 of 28 (7%) 100 mg: 4 of 28 (14%) 150 mg: 5 of 19 (26%) 300 mg: 4 of 20 (20%)	
	Treatment sequencing: NA	**Smoking characteristics:** Mean (SD) cigarettes/day range from 26.2 (8.5) to 27.5 (9.6)	12 mo rates for participants with history of MDD and alcohol dependence	
		Previous serious quit attempts range from 3.5 (3.4) to 4.3 (5.4)	Placebo: 1 of 3 (33%) 100 mg: 2 of 7 (28.6%) 150 mg: 4 of 7 (57%) 300 mg: 2 of 10 (20%)	
		FTND range from 7.1 (1.7) to 7.3 (1.7)		
		Comorbid conditions (n [%]): Lifetime alcohol dependence, n = 60		

Study ID: Hayford, Patten, Rummans, et al., 1999

Study Information	Interventions	Participant Characteristics	Results and Adverse Effects	Comments/ Quality Scoring
			2) Medication adherence rate: NR	
			3) Differential effects by gender: NR	
			4) Differential effects by depression status: NR	
			5) Differential effects by treatment sequencing: NA	
			Report adverse effects? Yes Discontinued due to AE: Placebo: 8 (5%) 100 mg: 9 (6%) 150 mg: 7 (5%) 300 mg: 13 (8%)	
			Headache, insomnia*, rhinitis, dry mouth*, and anxiety were most common (* = statistically significantly more)	
			Other: Among those continuously abstinent (n = 103), there was a dose x time interaction (p = 0.04) showing less weight gain as bupropion dose increased	

Comparative Effectiveness of Smoking Cessation Treatments
for Patients With Depression

Evidence-basedSynthesisProgram

Study ID: Kinnunen, Doherty, Militello, et al., 1996

Study Information	Interventions	Participant Characteristics	Results and Adverse Effects	Comments/ Quality Scoring
Geographical location: Boston, MA	**Intervention description:** Counseling + nicotine gum 2 mg vs counseling + nicotine gum 4 mg; combined gum (n = 178) vs counseling + placebo (n = 91)	**Inclusion criteria:** - Smoked ≥ 5 cigarettes/day - Good health - Age ≥ 20	**Follow-up rate:** NR	**General comments:** None
Recruitment: Advertisement	**Smoking cessation intervention:** _Behavioral interventions_	**Exclusion criteria:** NR	**Important baseline differences:** NR for intervention groups	**Applicability cautions:** - Mean age 40
Setting: NR	One-time brief individual behavioral counseling: behavioral-cognitive procedures for coping with urges, cravings and withdrawal symptoms; help with individual concerns about quitting, such as weight gain; no further information given	**Age:** Mean (SD)	Depressed patients were more likely to be female, older, and unmarried than the nondepressed	- > 50% female - > 80% white
Veterans clinics: No		Overall Depressed 40.4 (12.6) 41.6 (12.7)	**Outcomes of interest**	**Study-level quality assessment:** Good
Study design: Secondary analysis of RCT	_Drugs_ - Nicotine gum 2 mg ad lib; target usage of 9-15 pieces/day	**Gender (n [%]):** Female	**1) Abstinence rate:** Depressed subgroup (n = 93) at 90 days post–quit date:	**Measure of smoking adequate?**
Number of participants enrolled: 269 (93 depressed; 176 nondepressed)	- Nicotine gum 4 mg ad lib; target usage of 9-15 pieces/day	Overall Depressed 145 (51%) 56 (61%)	- Placebo: 4 of 33 (12.5%) - Nicotine gum 2 mg and 4 mg groups: 17 of 59 (29.5%)	Atypical definition; less stringent than other studies
Duration of follow-up: 3 mo post-quit date	**Depression intervention:** None	**Race/ethnicity (n [%]):** White	**2) Medication adherence rate:** Recommended gum use: 9 to 15 pieces/day	**Assessment of adverse effects adequate?** No; only assessed 7 day change in CES-D scores
Methods of assessment **Smoking status:** - History and expired CO - Relapse defined as "reestablished a regular pattern of smoking"; defined as ≥ 7 consecutive days	**Comparator intervention(s)** **Smoking cessation intervention:** _Behavioral interventions_ Same as intervention group	Overall Depressed 221 (82%) 74 (80%) Black Overall Depressed 29 (11%) 11 (12%) Other Overall Depressed 19 (7%) 8 (8%)	Average daily gum used for all groups at days 7, 30, 60, 90 was 8.1 pieces, 7.8 pieces, 6.2 pieces, 4.7 pieces, respectively **3) Differential effects by gender:** NR	
Depression status: CES-D score	_Drugs_ Matching placebo gum ad lib; target usage of 9-15 pieces/day Depression intervention: None Mean contact time/proportion of sessions completed: NR	**Baseline depression assessment:** CES-D, 20 items, 0-60	**4) Differential effects by depression status:** NR	
	Treatment sequencing: NA	**Smoking characteristics:** Mean cigarettes: 22 (10.4) Mean duration: 23.1 yr (4.0) FTND (depressed group): 5.6 (2.4)	**5) Differential effects by treatment sequencing:** NA **Report adverse effects?** - 7 day change in CES-D scores - Placebo group (depressed): no significant change, Tukey p = 0.99	
		Comorbid conditions: NR	- Nicotine group (depressed): lower scores, Tukey p = 0.00003	

62

Study ID: Kinnunen, Korhonen, and Garvey, 2008

Study Information	Interventions	Participant Characteristics	Results and Adverse Effects	Comments/ Quality Scoring
Geographical location: Boston, MA	**Intervention description:** - Nicotine gum, 2-4 mg (collapsed) (n = 405) - Placebo gum (n = 203)	**Inclusion criteria:** - Age ≥ 20 - Good health - Smoke ≥ 5 cigarettes/day	**Follow-up rate:** NR; 3 withdrew for adverse effects	**General comments:** Supplemented information using Garvey 2000
Recruitment: Advertisement	**Smoking cessation intervention:** _Behavioral interventions_ Individual brief (5-10 min) counseling at each in-person visit (1, 7, 14, 30, 60, 90, 180, 270, and 365 days post–quit date) Booklet "Clearing the Air" on how to stop smoking was provided	**Exclusion criteria:** - Serious medical condition - Use of psychiatric medications	**Important baseline differences:** Depressed group was younger, single, and had less education; $P < 0.05$	**Applicability cautions:** - Majority female - 80% White
Setting: - Clinic type NR - Academic (university hospital)		**Age:** Mean (SD) - NR for whole population - Depressed 38.5 (11.3) - Nondepressed 41.9 (12.0)	**Outcomes of interest** 1) **Abstinence rate:** - At 3 mo: In figure, but numbers not given; would have to extrapolate numbers	**Study-level quality assessment:** Good
Veterans clinics: No	**Drugs** NRT gum, 2 or 4 mg; groups collapsed across arms as parent study showed no difference in outcome between groups	**Gender (n [%]):** Female 312 (51%) Depressed female 110 (56.1%) Nondepressed female 202 (49%)	- At 12 mo: Nondepressed with NRT = 58 of 279 (20.1%) Nondepressed placebo = 20 of 133 (15.1%)	**Measure of smoking adequate?** Yes
Study design: RCT	**Depression intervention:** None		Depressed with NRT = 12 of 126 (9.8%) Depressed with placebo = 4/70 (5.7%)	**Assessment of adverse effects adequate?** Yes
Number of participants enrolled: Total n = 608 Depressed = 196 Nondepressed = 412	**Comparator intervention(s)** **Smoking cessation intervention:** _Behavioral interventions_ Individual brief (5-10 mi) counseling at each in-person visit Booklet "Clearing the Air" on how to stop smoking was provided	**Race/ethnicity (n [%]):** _Depressed_ _Nondepressed_ White 154 (78.6%) 338 (82%) Black 28 (14.3%) 51(12.4%) Other 14(7.1%) 23 (5.6%)	2) **Medication adherence rate:** NR	
Duration of follow-up: 3, 6, 9, and 12 mo post–quit date	**Drugs** Placebo gum	**Baseline depression assessment:** CES-D, range 0-60; ≥ 16 classified as depressed; 32% depressed at baseline	3) **Differential effects by gender:** NR, but effect of depression no longer significant when adjusted for differences in marital status and education	
Methods of assessment **Smoking status:** Self report 7-day point prevalence validated by CO monitor	**Depression intervention:** None	No information on history of depression or substance abuse	4) **Differential effects by depression status:** NR	
Depression status: CES-D score	**Mean contact time/proportion of sessions completed:** NR **Treatment sequencing:** NA	**Smoking characteristics:** - Expired CO > 8 ppm - Number of cigarettes/day - FTND	5) **Differential effects by treatment sequencing:** NR	
		Comorbid conditions (n [%]): Depression 195 (32%)	**Report adverse effects?** Yes 3 questionable reactions to NRT gum	

Comparative Effectiveness of Smoking Cessation Treatments for Patients With Depression

Study ID: MacPherson, Tull, Matusiewicz, et al., 2010

Study Information	Interventions	Participant Characteristics	Results and Adverse Effects	Comments/Quality Scoring
Geographical location: NR; multicenter?	**Intervention description:** 2 arms:	**Inclusion criteria:**	**Follow-up rate:** For abstinence obtained by bio-chemical verification of smoking status (others considered still smoking):	**General comments:** None
Recruitment: Advertisement	- ST: nicotine patch + 8 wk CBT (n = 33)	- Ages 18 to 65		**Applicability cautions:**
	- BATS: nicotine patch + 8 wk CBT + behavioral activation (BA) (n = 35)	- Smoke ≥ 10 cigarettes/day	Wk 1 78.6%	Age, gender, race, education and income all similar to veteran population
Setting:		- Smoke ≥ 1 yr	Wk 4 83.3%	
- Mental health, primary care, mixed	Matched for overall contact time; same specially trained therapists led both types of sessions; taped to ensure protocol followed (20% viewed)	- BDI-II ≥ 10	Wk 16 61.9%	**Study-level quality assessment:** Good
- Academic and nonacademic		- No current SCID-NP diagnosis	Wk 26 64.3%	
				Comments:
Veterans clinics: No	**Smoking cessation intervention:** Behavioral interventions	**Exclusion criteria:**	**Important baseline differences:** None (see Table 1)	- Repeated measures analyses using GEEs
Study design: RCT	30 min CBT (described in ST below, excluding relaxation; replaced with BA)	- BDI ≤ 7		- Random allocation
		- SCID Axis I diagnosis	**Outcomes of interest**	- Blinding not possible
Number of participants enrolled:	30 min of BA (adapted from Lejuez et al. 2001)	- Current use of psychotropic medications	1) Abstinence rate:	- Completers did not differ from ITT by demographics
- 68 randomized		- Current psychotherapy	ST BATS OR	
- 26 dropped out prior to treatment: 17 from standard treatment (ST); 9 from behavioral activation treatment for smoking (BATS)	Group therapy	- Contraindication to nicotine patch	ITT:	**Measure of smoking adequate?** Yes; only those whose smoking status was biochemically verified were considered abstinent at each time point, whereas the 26 missing participants who dropped out prior to treatment were considered as having smoked in ITT analyses
	Contact time 8 wk	- Use of smoking pharmacotherapy	Wk 16 3/33 4/35 2.71	
	Intervention delivered by psychology doctorate-level therapist	- Use of other types of tobacco	Wk 26 0/33 5/35 ---	
Duration of follow-up:			Completers:	
- 26 wk	Techniques specific to BA included activity monitoring (behavioral checkout form used for goal setting, planning, and monitoring throughout); identifying enjoyable activities and quit-related, abstinence-maintaining, and relapse-prevention activities	**Note: Demographics were not reported by entire population**	Wk 16 6.3 15.4 2.71	
- Measurements at baseline (wk 1), quit date (wk 4), 4 mo post–quit date (wk 16, but wk 12 post 8-wk treatment), and 6.5 mo post–quit date (wk 26, but wk 22 post 8-wk treatment)		**Age:**	Wk 26 0.0 19.2 ---	
	Drugs	Mean (SD)		
	Transdermal nicotine patch for 8 wk from quit date (wk 4) with an initial dose of 21 mg for 4 wk, followed by 14 mg for 2 wk, and 7 mg for 2 wk	ST BATS	Rates decreased over time, but interaction between treatment and time was ns	**Measure of smoking adequate?** Yes; only those whose smoking status was biochemically verified were considered abstinent at each time point, whereas the 26 missing participants who dropped out prior to treatment were considered as having smoked in ITT analyses
		42.6 (11.5) 45.0 (12.2)		
		Gender (n [%]):	BATS >ST (wk 1–wk 26 post–quit date)	
Methods of assessment	Participants who smoked on average 10-12 cigarettes/day started with the 14-mg patch for the first 6 wk per manufacturer's recommendations	Female:	abs OR 95% CI p	
Smoking status:		ST BATS	3.59 (1.22, 3.73) 0.02	
- 7 day self-reported point prevalence abstinence rates at 16 and 26 wk post-quit date	**Depression intervention:** Nothing additional to BA	16 (48.5%) 17 (48.6%)		
		Race/ethnicity (n [%]):	Continuous abstinence rates did not differ between treatments (p = 0.11)	**Assessment of adverse effects adequate?** NR
- Verified via expired CO		African American:		
- Saliva samples for cotinine analysis at wk 16 and 26		ST BATS	**Depression:** An interaction between treatment condition and the linear effect of time revealed that the reduction in depressive symptoms over time was greater for BATS than for ST participants (see Table 4, Figure 2)	
- Verification of abstinence defined as CO ≤10 ppm and cotinine ≤15 ng/ml		25 (75.8%) 24 (69.7%)		
		Baseline depression assessment: BDI, 0-62, score < or > 10:	This analysis is in completers (n =42)	
		ST BATS		
		10.4 (7.5) 10.8 (5.2)	BDI beta SE t p	
		Smoking characteristics:	-1.99 0.86 -2.31 0.02	
		FTND:		
		ST BATS		
		6.1 (2.1) 5.8 (1.8)		
		Cigarettes/day:		
		ST BATS		
		17.3 (8.1) 18.8 (7.1)		

Study ID: MacPherson, Tull, Matusiewicz, et al., 2010

Study Information	Interventions	Participant Characteristics	Results and Adverse Effects	Comments/ Quality Scoring
Depression status: BDI -II	**Comparator intervention(s)** **Smoking cessation intervention:** Behavioral interventions 60 min CBT Group therapy Contact time 8 sessions Intervention delivered by psychology doctorate-level therapist Techniques included self-monitoring, identifying effective and in-effective cessation strategies from prior quit attempts, relaxation, coping with triggers, identifying social support for cessation, making lifestyle changes (such as increasing physical activity and reducing stress), relapse prevention, and homework Drugs: Same as intervention **Depression intervention:** Behavioral interventions: None **Mean contact time/proportion of sessions completed:** ST: 11 of 16 completed 7 to 8 sessions BATS: 17 of 26 completed 7 to 8 sessions **Treatment sequencing:** NA **Other notes about interventions:** BA measured by Environmental Reward Observation Scale	**Comorbid conditions:** All were excluded	**2) Medication adherence rate:** See mean contact time **3) Differential effects by gender:** NR by treatment **4) Differential effects by de-pression status:** NR by treatment **5) Differential effects by treat-ment sequencing:** NA **Report adverse effects?** No List	

Comparative Effectiveness of Smoking Cessation Treatments for Patients With Depression

Study 1D: Munoz, Marin, Posner, et al, 1997

Study Information	Interventions	Participant Characteristics	Results and Adverse Effects	Comments/ Quality Scoring
Geographical location: San Francisco, CA	**Intervention description:** Mailed smoking cessation guide and mood management guide (immediate) vs smoking cessation guide and mood management guide at 3 mo (delayed)	**Inclusion criteria:** - Age 18+ - 3+ cigarettes/day - Completely or very sure they wanted to stop smoking within 3 mo - Able to read Spanish - Have access to audiotape player - Live in Bay area	**Follow-up rate:** Not clearly reported	**General comments:** Stratified randomization (no history of MDE vs history of or current MDE)
Recruitment: - TV - Radio - Newspaper - Bulletin boards - Health fairs	Immediate vs delayed: N = 71 (54 MDE) vs n = 65 (52 MDE) Incentives: - $2 for each 2 wk chart up to 6 charts in mood management - $10 for each assessment a 3 mo and 6 mo - $10 for saliva sample	**Exclusion criteria:** None	**Important baseline differences:** Delayed group had lower education and was less likely to be employed	**Applicability cautions;** Spanish speaking only
Setting: Community		**Age:** Mean (SD): 35.3, SD = NR	**Outcomes of interest** 1) Abstinence rate: (by self report)	**Study-level quality assessment:** Fair
Veterans clinics: No	**Smoking cessation intervention:** Behavioral interventions	**Gender (n [%]):** Women 52 (38.2%) Men 84 (61.8%)	Immediate (3 mo) No MDE .... 4 of 17 Current .... 4 of 28 MDE history .... 8 of 26	**Comments:** - Randomization and allocation concealment procedures not well described - No assessment of cotreatments (e.g., NRT)
Study design: RCT	The "GUIA" (Guia Para Dejar de Fumar), a 36-page brochure published in Spanish NCI (2002), is an anti-smoking brochure published in Spanish that includes reasons to quit, preparing to quit, techniques to resist the urge to smoke as a result of social situations, and changes in diet and exercise to avoid weight gain	**Race/ethnicity (n [%]):** Latino 136 (100%)	Immediate (6 mo) No MDE .... 3 of 17 Current .... 5 of 28 MDE history .... 10 of 26	
Number of participants enrolled: 136		**Baseline depression assessment:** Modified DIS CES-D for level of depressive symptoms	Delayed (3 mo) No MDE .... 1 of 13 Current .... 3 of 25 MDE history .... 3 of 27	- Follow-up rates not clearly reported - Biochemical verification done, but results not reported
Duration of follow-up: 3 mo, 6 mo				**Measure of smoking adequate?** Yes; but not clearly reported
Methods of assessment	Mood management intervention, "Tomando Control de Su Vida," an audio cassette on how to use materials, 30-minute relaxation exercise, self-monitoring of cigarette use booklet, pleasant activity guide, and monitoring tool		Delayed (6 mo) No MDE .... 2 of 13 Current .... 2 of 25 MDE history .... 2 of 27	**Assessment of adverse effects adequate?** NA
Smoking status: Self-report of 7 day abstinence from cigarettes using mailed self-monitoring charts; saliva cotinine using 14 ng/ml as cut point but results not reported using this method	A call was placed to verify receipt of materials and answer questions Drugs: None		**2) Medication adherence rate:** Not clearly reported Those returning filled out materials in immediate group vs those that did not = 45% vs 14% abstinence at 3 mo	
	Depression intervention: None (note that we have classified the mood management module as part of the smoking cessation intervention, but it could be classified as a depression intervention)	**Immediate:** 21.5 (14.9) **Delayed:** 20.7 (12.5) Lifetime MDE n = 106 Current = 53 History = 53 No MDE history = 30	**3) Differential effects by gender:** NR	
	Comparator intervention(s) Smoking cessation intervention: Behavioral interventions GUIA plus delayed (3 mo) mood management; essentially a waitlist control	**Smoking characteristics:** Number of cigarettes/day 14.1 (8.2)	**4) Differential effects by depression status:** See above for unadjusted results	
Depression status: CES-D	Drugs: None Depression intervention: None Mean contact time/proportion of sessions completed: NR Treatment sequencing: NA	**Comorbid conditions:** NR	**5) Differential effects by treatment sequencing:** NA **Report adverse effects?** NR	

Comparative Effectiveness of Smoking Cessation Treatments for Patients With Depression

Evidence-basedSynthesisProgram

Study 1D: Saules, Schuh, Arfken, et al., 2004

Study Information	Interventions	Participant Characteristics	Results and Adverse Effects	Comments/ Quality Scoring

Geographical location: NR; multisite?
 	
Recruitment: Advertisement
 	
Setting:
- Mental health clinic
- Academic
 	
Veterans clinics: No
 	
Study design: RCT
 	
Number of participants enrolled: 150
 	
Duration of follow-up: 3, 6, and 12 mo post-quit date
 	
Methods of assessment
Smoking status: Nonsmoking defined as self-reported abstinence combined with CO < 10 ppm
Depression status: BDI
	Intervention description: 3-arm study investigated the addition of fluoxetine to standard treatment to improve smoking cessation in smokers with depression:
	
	Fluoxetine (20 mg) + NRT + CBT (n = 48)
	Fluoxetine (40 mg) + NRT + CBT (n = 51)
	Placebo + NRT + CBT (n = 51)
	
	Smoking cessation intervention:
	Behavioral interventions
	6 wk of group CBT started 2 wk prior to quit date delivered by trained therapists with treatment manual; no further information given
	
	Drugs
	- 14 wk of either 20 mg or 40 mg of fluoxetine started 4 wk before quit date
	- 10 wk of standard (15 mg dose) transdermal NRT started at quit date; 6 wk on 15 mg, then 2 wk 10 mg, and 2 wk 5 mg
	
	Depression intervention:
	Behavioral interventions
	Nothing in addition to standard CBT (fluoxetine is an antidepressant, however)
	
	Comparator intervention(s)
	Smoking cessation intervention:
	Behavioral interventions
	Same as intervention group
	
	Drugs
	- 14 wk of placebo started 4 wk before quit date
	- Standard transdermal patch NRT as above
	
	Depression intervention:
	Behavioral interventions
	Same as intervention; nothing in addition to standard CBT
	
	Mean contact time/proportion of sessions completed:
	60% completed active phase; no difference between groups
	
	Treatment sequencing: NA
		Inclusion criteria:
		- Ages 21 to 65
		- $\geq$ 15 cigarettes/day
		- Expired CO $\geq$ 15 ppm
		
		Exclusion criteria:
		- Psychiatric episode in last 6 mo
		- Current psychiatric medication use
		- Pregnancy
		- Poor comprehension
		- Any clinically significant medical condition
		
		Age:
		Total pop (mean) 39.78
		SDs NR
		Range: 21 to 65
		   Placebo 20mg 40mg
		   40.85 40.44 38.44
		
		Gender (n [%]):
		Female:
		  Placebo 20mg 40mg
		 23 (44.7%) 31(60.8%) 27(56.9%)
		
		Race/ethnicity (n [%]):
		White:
		 Placebo 20mg 40mg
		 78.3% 74.5% 67.3%
		
		Black:
		 Placebo 20mg 40mg
		 21.7% 21.3% 26.5%
		
		Other:
		 Placebo 20mg 40mg
		 --- 4.2% 6.2%
		
		Baseline depression assessment:
		BDI (mean score):
		 Placebo 20 mg 40 mg
		 6.34 5.14 3.33
		
		Smoking characteristics:
		FTND (score);
		 Placebo 20 mg 40 mg
		 6.13 6.08 5.51
		
		Comorbid conditions (n [%]):
		History of MDD (%)
		 Placebo 20 mg 40 mg
		 17.0% 22.0% 22.0%
		
		State-Trait Anxiety (%)
		 Placebo 20 mg 40 mg
		 43.69% 46.29% 44.50%
			Follow-up rate:
			Follow-up rates NR for 3, 6, 12 mo follow-ups
			
			Important baseline differences:
			Higher BDI in placebo group; $F(2,129) = 3.39$, $p = 0.037$
			
			Outcomes of interest
			At 15 wk from start of study, smoking cessation = 40%
			
			1) Abstinence rate:
			At 15 wk:
			Total (n = 150)
			Placebo = 35.4%
			20 mg fluoxetine = 43.1%
			40 mg fluoxetine = 43.1%
			
			History of MDD (n = 30)
			Placebo = 37.5%
			20 mg fluoxetine = 54.5%
			40 mg fluoxetine = 54.5%
			But these n's are small ~ 10
			
			2) Medication adherence: NR
			
			3) Differential effects by gender: None
			
			4) Differential effects by depression status: None
			
			5) Differential effects by treatment sequencing: NA
			
			Report adverse effects? Yes; but only that they were lower in both fluoxetine groups compared to placebo ($p = 0.038$) using the Minnesota Tobacco Withdrawal Symptom Checklist
				General comments:
				Population not depressed (BDI score = 4.92 and only 20% had a history of depression), but results given by whether or not history of MDD was present
				
				Subjects were paid $25 to complete, $150 for follow-up, and $50 at final visit
				
				Applicability cautions:
				College educated, mean = 79.3%
				
				Study-level quality assessment: Fair
				
				Comments:
				- No rates of treatment discontinuation by arm
				- Selective outcome reporting: Did not report smoking rates by arm across 3, 6, 12 mo follow-ups.
				- Did not report loss to follow-up
				
				Measure of smoking adequate? Yes; cotinine
				
				Assessment of adverse effects adequate? Assessment method not given; reported that number of AEs did not differ between groups

67

Study ID: Vickers, Patten, Lewis, et al., 2009

Study Information	Interventions	Participant Characteristics	Results and Adverse Effects	Comments/ Quality Scoring
Geographical location: Rochester, MN	**Intervention description:** Tested addition of exercise to NRT in a depressed female population to aid smoking abstinence	**Inclusion criteria:** - Female - Ages 18 to 65 - CES-D ≥ 16 - Cigarettes ≥ 10/day for past 6 mo - Current exercise < 20 min on fewer than 3 day/wk - Ability to do exercise - Good health - Negative pregnancy test - BMI ≤ 40	**There were no significant differences between groups on any outcome variable**	**General comments:** Subjects were paid a nominal fee: $25 at end of treatment (wk 10) and $25 after follow-up (wk 24)
Recruitment: Advertisement	Intervention: NRT + exercise + smoking cessation behavioral counseling (n = 30)		**Follow-up rate:** Wk 24 follow-up: Treatment Control 16 of 30 (53%) 15 of 30 (50%)	
Setting: - Mental health, primary care, mixed - Academic and nonacademic	Control: NRT + health education + smoking cessation behavioral counseling (n = 30)		**Important baseline differences:** Current psychotherapy: Treatment Control 7 (23) 11 (37)	**Applicability cautions:** - 65% college-educated - 100% overweight white females
Veterans clinics: No	**Smoking cessation intervention:** Behavioral interventions Brief smoking cessation counseling (10 min/visit) with handouts and NCI "Clearing the Air" brochure via same specialist as CBT for exercise	**Exclusion criteria:** - Recent MI - Substance abuse - Psychosis - Nortriptyline, bupropion - Other tobacco product use - Skin allergies or other problems with NRT patch - Suicidal ideation	Current pharmacotherapy: Treatment Control 16 (53) 19 (63)	**Study-level quality assessment:** Fair to poor
Study design: RCT			**Outcomes of interest** 1) Abstinence rate: Wk 24 follow-up Treatment Control 1 of 16 (6.3%) 1 of 15 (6.7%)	**Comments:** - Small pilot, not powered for any statistical test stronger than analysis via 2 sample, rank-sum test
Number of participants enrolled: 60	**Drugs** Transdermal patch NRT (21 mg/day) started on quit date (wk 4), continued through wk 10		2) Medication adherence rate: NRT: Treatment Control 36% 31%	- In the exercise literature, not helping overweight people with the actual exercise has been shown to be of no benefit
Duration of follow-up: End of treatment = 10 wk Follow-up = 24 wk	**Depression intervention:** Behavioral interventions 10 wk social cognitive theory–informed CBT exercise intervention strategies (not actual exercise) to encourage patient to meet the CDC/ACSM 1995 guidelines of moderate physical activity (30 min/day x 5 wk) via trained (manual and observation) patient education specialist via ten 30 min weekly sessions	**Age:** Range: 18 to 65 Mean (SD): Treatment Control 40.9 (11.8) 41.8 (12.1)	Exercise or Education: Treatment Control 49% 21%	- Missing outcome data on 50% of sample by wk24
Methods of assessment Smoking status: Self-reported, 7-day point prevalence abstinence verified by expired CO < 8 ppm at end of treatment and urine cotinine at follow-up wk 24	Topics included benefits, goal setting, reinforcement, problem solving, overcoming barriers, and relapse prevention Exercise activity was self-monitored.	**Gender (n [%]):** Female 60 (100%)	**3) Differential effects by gender:** NA (all female)	**Measure of smoking adequate?** Yes
Depression status: HSRD	**Comparator intervention(s) Smoking cessation intervention:** Behavioral interventions Same as intervention (above); brief counseling (10 min/visit) with handouts via same specialist as health education	**Race/ethnicity (n [%]):** White 59 (98%) - Black 1 (2%) in exercise group - White 30 (100%) in control group	**4) Differential effects by depression status:** NR	**Assessment of adverse effects adequate?** NR
	Drugs: Same as intervention	**Baseline depression assessment:** CES-D, 0-60, > 16 Treatment Control 29.8(9.3) 32.4(9.6)	**5) Differential effects by treatment sequencing:** NA	
	Depression intervention: Behavioral interventions Equal time/contact control using health education via patient education specialist; topics included sleep, nutrition, preventive screening tests	HRSD Treatment Control 12.8(6.0) 15.4(9.3)	**Report adverse effects?** No	
	Mean contact time/proportion of sessions completed: Mean (SD) sessions completed out of 10 sessions: Treatment Control 7.6(3.5) 8.2(2.7)			

Comparative Effectiveness of Smoking Cessation Treatments for Patients With Depression

Study ID: Vickers, Patten, Lewis, et al., 2009

Study Information	Interventions	Participant Characteristics	Results and Adverse Effects	Comments/ Quality Scoring
	Treatment sequencing: NA	**Smoking characteristics:**		
		Cigarettes/day:		
	Other notes about interventions:	Treatment Control		
	- Important to note that subjects were left on their own to find venues and types of actual exercise	20.0 (7.8) 21.6 (7.3)		
		FTND score ≥ 6		
	- Also measured weight, weight concerns, change in mood (Positive and Negative Affect Scale), fitness level (VO2 max test), and physical activity (physical activity recall)	Treatment Control		
		16 (53) 20 (67)		
		Comorbid conditions (n [%]):		
		None medical or psychiatric; all excluded		
		but examined weight concern:		
		Treatment Control		
		5.8 (2.2%) 6.6 (2.1%)		
		Weight, kg:		
		Treatment Control		
		76.0 (15.1%) 73.6 (15.7%)		

Abbreviations: AE = adverse effects, am = ante meridian (before noon), BA = behavioral activation, BATS = behavioral activation treatment for smoking, BDI-II = Beck Depression Inventory–II, BID = two times per day, CBT = cognitive behavioral therapy, CES-D = Center for Epidemiologic Studies-Depression Scale, CI = confidence interval, CO = carbon monoxide, DIS = Diagnostic Interview Schedule, FTND = Fagerstrom Test for Nicotine Dependence, GEE = generalized estimating equation, HDRS = Hamilton Depression Rating Scale, ID = identification, ITT = intention to treat, MDD = major depressive disorder, MDE = major depressive episode, mg = milligram or milligrams, ml = milliliter, mo = month/months, n = number, NA = not applicable, NCI = National Cancer Institute, ng = nanogram, NR = not reported, NRT = nicotine replacement therapy, ns = not significant, OR = odds ratio, p = probability, pm = post meridian (afternoon), POMS = Profile of Mood States, ppm = parts per million, RCT = randomized controlled trial, SCID = Structured Clinical Interview for DSM Diagnoses, SD = standard deviation, SE = standard error, ST = standard treatment, UDD = unipolar depressive disorder, vs = versus, wk = week/weeks, yr = year/years

LIST OF INCLUDED STUDIES IN ALPHABETICAL ORDER

Brown RA, Kahler CW, Niaura R, et al. Cognitive-behavioral treatment for depression in smoking cessation. J Consult Clin Psychol 2001;69(3):471-80.

Covey LS, Glassman AH, Stetner F. Naltrexone effects on short-term and long-term smoking cessation. J Addict Dis 1999;18(1):31-40.

Covey LS, Glassman AH, Stetner F, et al. A randomized trial of sertraline as a cessation aid for smokers with a history of major depression. Am J Psychiatry 2002;159(10):1731-7.

Duffy SA, Ronis DL, Valenstein M, et al. A tailored smoking, alcohol, and depression intervention for head and neck cancer patients. Cancer Epidemiol Biomarkers Prev 2006;15(11):2203-8.

Evins AE, Culhane MA, Alpert JE, et al. A controlled trial of bupropion added to nicotine patch and behavioral therapy for smoking cessation in adults with unipolar depressive disorders. J Clin Psychopharmacol 2008;28(6):660-6.

Hall SM, Munoz RF, Reus VI. Cognitive-behavioral intervention increases abstinence rates for depressive-history smokers. J Consult Clin Psychol 1994;62(1):141-6.

Hall SM, Munoz RF, Reus VI, et al. Mood management and nicotine gum in smoking treatment: a therapeutic contact and placebo-controlled study. J Consult Clin Psychol 1996;64(5):1003-9.

Hall SM, Reus VI, Munoz RF, et al. Nortriptyline and cognitive-behavioral therapy in the treatment of cigarette smoking. Arch Gen Psychiatry 1998;55(8):683-90.

Hall SM, Tsoh JY, Prochaska JJ, et al. Treatment for cigarette smoking among depressed mental health outpatients: a randomized clinical trial. Am J Public Health 2006;96(10):1808-14.

Hayford KE, Patten CA, Rummans TA, et al. Efficacy of bupropion for smoking cessation in smokers with a former history of major depression or alcoholism. Br J Psychiatry 1999;174:173-8.

Kinnunen T, Doherty K, Militello FS, et al. Depression and smoking cessation: characteristics of depressed smokers and effects of nicotine replacement. J Consult Clin Psychol 1996;64(4):791-8.

Kinnunen T, Korhonen T, Garvey AJ. Role of nicotine gum and pretreatment depressive symptoms in smoking cessation: twelve-month results of a randomized placebo controlled trial. Int J Psychiatry Med 2008;38(3):373-89.

MacPherson L, Tull MT, Matusiewicz AK, et al. Randomized controlled trial of behavioral activation smoking cessation treatment for smokers with elevated depressive symptoms. J Consult Clin Psychol 2010;78(1):55-61.

Munoz RF, Marin BV, Posner SF, et al. Mood management mail intervention increases abstinence rates for Spanish-speaking Latino smokers. Am J Community Psychol 1997;25(3):325-43.

Saules KK, Schuh LM, Arfken CL, et al. Double-blind placebo-controlled trial of fluoxetine in smoking cessation treatment including nicotine patch and cognitive-behavioral group therapy. Am J Addict 2004;13(5):438-46.

Vickers KS, Patten CA, Lewis BA, et al. Feasibility of an exercise counseling intervention for depressed women smokers. Nicotine Tob Res 2009;11(8):985-95.

APPENDIX D: EXCLUDED STUDIES

All studies listed in Table 12 were reviewed in their full-text version and excluded for the reason indicated. An alphabetical reference list follows the table.

Table 12. List of Excluded Studies

Reference	Population not depressed	Main outcome not of interest to key questions	Not peer-reviewed	Main outcome not reported at desired interval	Not RCT or secondary analysis	Analysis does not address key questions
Acton, 2005 (203)	X					
Alderton, 2009 (5)					X	
Barnett, 2008 (82)		X				
Bercaw, 2008 (963)			X			
Berlin, 2006 (141)				X		
Blondal, 1999 (1317)						X
Brown, 2007 (117)	X					
Buchanan, 2004 (1247)	X					
Capone, 2003 (968)			X			
Carmody, 2008 (567)	X					
Carton, 2002 (300)	X					
Catley, 2003 (278)	X					
Catley, 2005 (179)	X					
Collins, 2003 (1265)			X			
Cornelius, 1997 (1036)		X				
Covey, 2008 (1204)	X					
Covey, 1990 (445)				X		
Cox, 2004 (237)		X				
Csonka, 2008 (1206)			X			
Dalack, 1995 (413)		X				
Frederick, 1996 (924)		X				
Friend, 2007 (123)	X					
Gilbert,1999 (366)		X				

Comparative Effectiveness of Smoking Cessation Treatments for Patients With Depression

Reference	Population not depressed	Main outcome not of interest to key questions	Not peer-reviewed	Main outcome not reported at desired interval	Not RCT or secondary analysis	Analysis does not address key questions
Ginsberg, 1995 (1086)		X				
Ginsberg, 1997 (381)		X				
Glassman, 1993 (425)	X					
Glassman, 2001 (325)		X				
Glassman, 1988 (451)				X		
Haas, 2005 (235)						X
Hayford, 1997 (1325)			X			
Helgason, 2004 (742)					X	
Hernandez-Reif, 1999 (369)	X					
Hill, 2007 (626)					X	
Hitsman,1999 (363)	X					
Jarvik, 2000 (1297)	X					
Keuthen, 2000 (343)	X					
Killen,1999 (1035)	X					
Killen, 2008 (1197)	X					X
Lerman, 2004A (1256)	X					
Lerman, 2004 B(215)		X				
Leventhal, 2008 (85)	X					
Levine, 2000 (1152)			X		X	
McCarthy, 2008 (587)	X					
McClure, 2009 (34)						X
McFall, 2005 (1240)	X					
McHugh, 2001 (1291)	X					
Mermelstein, 2003 (788)	X					
Munoz, 2006 (165)						X
Oncken, 2007 (641)	X					
Patten, 2002 (304)				X		
Patten, 1998 (375)	X					
Perkins, 2008 (1199)		X				

Comparative Effectiveness of Smoking Cessation Treatments
for Patients With Depression

Reference	Population not depressed	Main outcome not of interest to key questions	Not peer-reviewed	Main outcome not reported at desired interval	Not RCT or secondary analysis	Analysis does not address key questions
Piper, 2010 (1113)	X					
Pomerleau, 2003 (2854)		X				
Prochaska, 2008 (115)		X				
Rabius, 2008 (42)	X					
Rovina, 2007 (604)					X	
Schippers, 2006 (1233)				X		
Smith, 2003 (276)	X					
Sonne, 2010 (465)	X					
Spring, 2007A (133)				X		
Spring, 2004 (1255)						
Spring, 2007B (150)					X	
Strong, 2009 (8)	X					
Swan, 2003 (772)	X					
Thorndike, 2008 (91)	X					
Thorndike, 2006 (1228)	X					
Trockel, 2008 (53)	X					
Uyar, 2007 (607)	X					
Vazquez, 1999 (357)					X	
Walsh, 2008 (74)	X					
Wetter, 1999 (884)	X					
Wileyto, 2005 (189)		X				
Zelman, 1992 (946)	X					
Ziedonis, 1997 (1328)	X					

LIST OF EXCLUDED STUDIES

Acton GS, Kunz JD, Wilson M, et al. The construct of internalization: conceptualization, measurement, and prediction of smoking treatment outcome. Psychol Med 2005;35(3):395-408.

Alderton W, Karran E, Ward S. Current and Future Perspectives in Psychiatric Drug Discovery. Drug News Perspect 2009;22(6):360-4.

Barnett PG, Wong W, Hall S. The cost-effectiveness of a smoking cessation program for outpatients in treatment for depression. Addiction 2008;103(5):834-40.

Bercaw EL. A behavioral activation approach to smoking cessation for depressed smokers at veterans affairs medical centers. ProQuest Information & Learning; 2008.

Berlin I, Covey LS. Pre-cessation depressive mood predicts failure to quit smoking: the role of coping and personality traits. Addiction 2006;101(12):1814-21.

Blondal T, Gudmundsson LJ, Tomasson K, et al. The effects of fluoxetine combined with nicotine inhalers in smoking cessation--a randomized trial. Addiction (Abingdon, England) 1999(7):1007-15.

Brown RA, Niaura R, Lloyd-Richardson EE, et al. Bupropion and cognitive-behavioral treatment for depression in smoking cessation. Nicotine Tob Res 2007;9(7):721-30.

Buchanan LM, El-Banna M, White A, et al. An exploratory study of multicomponent treatment intervention for tobacco dependency. Journal of nursing scholarship : an official publication of Sigma Theta Tau International Honor Society of Nursing / Sigma Theta Tau 2004(4):324-30.

Capone D-AL. An emotion-focused problem-solving smoking cessation intervention for depression-prone college students. ProQuest Information & Learning; 2003.

Carmody TP, Duncan C, Simon JA, et al. Hypnosis for smoking cessation: A randomized trial. Nicotine Tob Res 2008;10(5):811-818.

Carton S, Le Houezec J, Lagrue G, et al. Early emotional disturbances during nicotine patch therapy in subjects with and without a history of depression. J Affect Disord 2002;72(2):195-9.

Catley D, Ahluwalia JS, Resnicow K, et al. Depressive symptoms and smoking cessation among inner-city African Americans using the nicotine patch. Nicotine Tob Res 2003;5(1):61-8.

Catley D, Harris KJ, Okuyemi KS, et al. The influence of depressive symptoms on smoking cessation among African Americans in a randomized trial of bupropion. Nicotine Tob Res 2005;7(6):859-70.

Collins BN, Niaura R, Wileyto EP, et al. Effect of bupropion on depression symptoms in highly dependent smokers. Society for Research on Nicotine and Tobacco 9th Annual Meeting February 19-22 New Orleans, LA 2003:98.

Cornelius JR, Salloum Ihsan M, Ehler JG, et al. Double-blind fluoxetine in depressed alcoholic smokers. Psychopharmacol Bull 1997;33(1):165-170.

Covey LS, Botello-Harbaum M, Glassman AH, et al. Smokers' response to combination bupropion, nicotine patch, and counseling treatment by race/ethnicity. Ethn Dis 2008(1):59-64.

Covey LS, Glassman AH, Stetner F. Depression and depressive symptoms in smoking cessation. Compr Psychiatry 1990;31(4):350-4.

Cox LS, Patten CA, Niaura RS, et al. Efficacy of bupropion for relapse prevention in smokers with and without a past history of major depression. J Gen Intern Med 2004;19(8):828-34.

Csonka A, Jonas Z. The combination of targeted cognitive-behavioural psychotherapy and pharmacotherapy for patients suffering from depression in smoking cessation. International Journal of Neuropsychopharmacology 2008(Suppl. 1):92.

Dalack GW, Glassman AH, Rivelli S, et al. Mood, major depression, and fluoxetine response in cigarette smokers. Am J Psychiatry 1995;152(3):398-403.

Frederick SL, Humfleet GL, Hall SM, et al. Sex differences in the relation of mood to weight gain after quitting smoking. Experimental and Clinical Psychopharmacology 1996;4(2):178-185.

Friend KB, Pagano ME. Timevarying predictors of smoking cessation among individuals in treatment for alcohol abuse and dependence: findings from Project MATCH. Alcohol Alcohol 2007;42(3):234-40.

Gilbert DG, Crauthers DM, Mooney DK, et al. Effects of monetary contingencies on smoking relapse: influences of trait depression, personality, and habitual nicotine intake. Exp Clin Psychopharmacol 1999;7(2):174-81.

Ginsberg D, Hall SM, Reus VI, et al. Mood and depression diagnosis in smoking cessation. Experimental and Clinical Psychopharmacology 1995;3(4):389-395.

Ginsberg JP, Klesges RC, Johnson KC, et al. The relationship between a history of depression and adherence to a multicomponent smoking-cessation program. Addict Behav 1997;22(6):783-7.

Glassman AH, Covey LS, Dalack GW, et al. Smoking cessation, clonidine, and vulnerability to nicotine among dependent smokers. Clin Pharmacol Ther 1993;54(6):670-9.

Glassman AH, Covey LS, Stetner F, et al. Smoking cessation and the course of major depression: a follow-up study. Lancet 2001;357(9272):1929-32.

Glassman AH, Stetner F, Walsh BT, et al. Heavy smokers, smoking cessation, and clonidine. Results of a double-blind, randomized trial. JAMA 1988;259(19):2863-6.

Haas AL, Munoz RF, Humfleet GL, et al. Influences of mood, depression history, and treatment modality on outcomes in smoking cessation. J Consult Clin Psychol 2004;72(4):563-70.

Hayford KE, Patten CA, Rummans TA, et al. Effectiveness of Bupropion for Smoking Cessation for Smokers with a History of Major Depression CONFERENCE ABSTRACT. 150th Annual Meeting of the American Psychiatric Association. San Diego, California, USA. 17-22 May, 1997. 1997.

Helgason AR, Tomson T, Lund KE, et al. Factors related to abstinence in a telephone helpline for smoking cessation. European Journal of Public Health 2004;14(3):306-310.

Hernandez-Reif M, Field T, Hart S. Smoking cravings are reduced by self-massage. Prev Med 1999;28(1):28-32.

Hill KP, Chang G. Cognitive behavioral therapy and nicotine replacement for smoking cessation in psychiatric outpatients with major depression. Addictive Disorders and their Treatment 2007;6(2):67-72.

Hitsman B, Pingitore R, Spring B, et al. Antidepressant pharmacotherapy helps some cigarette smokers more than others. J Consult Clin Psychol 1999;67(4):547-54.

Jarvik ME, Caskey NH, Wirshing WC, et al. Bromocriptine reduces cigarette smoking. Addiction (Abingdon, England) 2000(8):1173-83.

Keuthen NJ, Niaura RS, Borrelli B, et al. Comorbidity, smoking behavior and treatment outcome. Psychother Psychosom 2000;69(5):244-50.

Killen JD, Fortmann SP, Davis L, et al. Do heavy smokers benefit from higher dose nicotine patch therapy? Experimental and Clinical Psychopharmacology 1999;7(3):226-233.

Killen JD, Fortmann SP, Schatzberg AF, et al. Extended cognitive behavior therapy for cigarette smoking cessation. Addiction (Abingdon, England) 2008(8):1381-90.

Lerman C, Kaufmann V, Rukstalis M, et al. Individualizing nicotine replacement therapy for the treatment of tobacco dependence: a randomized trial. *Ann Intern Med*; 2004:426-33. (A)

Lerman C, Niaura R, Collins BN, et al. Effect of bupropion on depression symptoms in a smoking cessation clinical trial. Psychol Addict Behav 2004;18(4):362-6. (B)

Leventhal AM, Ramsey SE, Brown RA, et al. Dimensions of depressive symptoms and smoking cessation. Nicotine Tob Res 2008;10(3):507-17.

Levine MD. The effect of depression history on smoking cessation in weight-concerned women. ProQuest Information & Learning; 2000.

McCarthy DE, Piasecki TM, Lawrence DL, et al. A randomized controlled clinical trial of bupropion SR and individual smoking cessation counseling. Nicotine Tob Res 2008;10(4):717-729.

McClure JB, Swan GE, Jack L, et al. Mood, side-effects and smoking outcomes among persons with and without probable lifetime depression taking varenicline. J Gen Intern Med 2009;24(5):563-9.

McFall M, Saxon AJ, Thompson CE, et al. Improving the rates of quitting smoking for veterans with posttraumatic stress disorder. The American Journal of Psychiatry 2005(7):1311-9.

McHugh F, Lindsay GM, Hanlon P, et al. Nurse led shared care for patients on the waiting list for coronary artery bypass surgery: a randomised controlled trial. Heart (British Cardiac Society) 2001(3):317-23.

Mermelstein R, Hedeker D, Wong SC. Extended telephone counseling for smoking cessation: Does content matter? J Consult Clin Psychol 2003;71(3):565-574.

Munoz RF, Lenert LL, Delucchi K, et al. Toward evidence-based Internet interventions: A Spanish/English Web site for international smoking cessation trials. Nicotine Tob Res 2006;8(1):77-87.

Oncken C, Cooney J, Feinn R, et al. Transdermal nicotine for smoking cessation in postmenopausal women. Addict Behav 2007;32(2):296-309.

Patten CA, Drews AA, Myers MG, et al. Effect of depressive symptoms on smoking abstinence and treatment adherence among smokers with a history of alcohol dependence. Psychol Addict Behav 2002;16(2):135-42.

Patten CA, Martin JE, Myers MG, et al. Effectiveness of cognitive-behavioral therapy for smokers with histories of alcohol dependence and depression. J Stud Alcohol 1998;59(3):327-35.

Perkins KA, Ciccocioppo M, Conklin CA, et al. Mood influences on acute smoking responses are independent of nicotine intake and dose expectancy. J Abnorm Psychol 2008(1):79-93.

Piper ME, Smith SS, Schlam TR, et al. Psychiatric disorders in smokers seeking treatment for tobacco dependence: Relations with tobacco dependence and cessation. J Consult Clin Psychol 2010;78(1):13-23.

Pomerleau OF, Pomerleau CS, Marks JL, et al. Prolonged nicotine patch use in quitters with past abstinence-induced depressed mood. J Subst Abuse Treat 2003;24(1):13-8.

Prochaska JJ, Hall SM, Tsoh JY, et al. Treating tobacco dependence in clinically depressed smokers: effect of smoking cessation on mental health functioning. Am J Public Health 2008;98(3):446-8.

Rabius V, Pike KJ, Wiatrek D, et al. Comparing internet assistance for smoking cessation: 13-month follow-up of a six-arm randomized controlled trial. J Med Internet Res 2008;10(5):e45.

Rovina N, Nikoloutsou I, Dima E, et al. Smoking cessation treatment in a real-life setting: The Greek experience. Therapeutic Advances in Respiratory Disease 2007;1(2):93-104.

Schippers G, Van der Meer R, Willemsen M, et al. Preliminary results from a RCT of a smoking cessation intervention for smokers with a history of major depression. Eur Neuropsychopharmacol 2006:S201.

Smith SS, Jorenby DE, Leischow SJ, et al. Targeting smokers at increased risk for relapse: treating women and those with a history of depression. Nicotine Tob Res 2003;5(1):99-109.

Sonne SC, Nunes EV, Jiang H, et al. The relationship between depression and smoking cessation outcomes in treatment-seeking substance abusers. Am J Addict 2010;19(2):111-118.

Spring B, Doran N, Pagoto S, et al. Fluoxetine, smoking, and history of major depression: A randomized controlled trial. J Consult Clin Psychol 2007;75(1):85-94. (A)

Spring B, Hines E. Fluoxetine as a quit smoking aid for depression-prone smokers. ClinicalTrials.gov. Available at: www.clinicaltrials.gov 2004.

Spring B, Hitsman B, Pingitore R, et al. Effect of tryptophan depletion on smokers and nonsmokers with and without history of major depression. Biol Psychiatry 2007;61(1):70-7. (B)

Strong DR, Kahler CW, Leventhal AM, et al. Impact of bupropion and cognitive-behavioral treatment for depression on positive affect, negative affect, and urges to smoke during cessation treatment. Nicotine Tob Res 2009;11(10):1142-53.

Swan GE, Jack LM, Curry S, et al. Bupropion SR and counseling for smoking cessation in actual practice: Predictors of outcome. Nicotine Tob Res 2003;5(6):911-921.

Thorndike AN, Regan S, McKool K, et al. Depressive symptoms and smoking cessation after hospitalization for cardiovascular disease. Arch Intern Med 2008;168(2):186-91.

Thorndike FP, Friedman-Wheeler DG, Haaga DA. Effect of cognitive behavior therapy on smokers' compensatory coping skills. Addict Behav 2006(9):1705-10.

Trockel M, Burg M, Jaffe A, et al. Smoking behavior postmyocardial infarction among ENRICHD trial participants: cognitive behavior therapy intervention for depression and low perceived social support compared with care as usual. Psychosom Med 2008;70(8):875-82.

Uyar M, Filiz A, Bayram N, et al. A randomized trial of smoking cessation. Medication versus motivation. Saudi Medical Journal 2007;28(6):922-926.

Vazquez FL, Becona E. Depression and smoking in a smoking cessation programme. J Affect Disord 1999;55(2-3):125-32.

Walsh Z, Epstein A, Munisamy G, et al. The impact of depressive symptoms on the efficacy of naltrexone in smoking cessation. J Addict Dis 2008;27(1):65-72.

Wetter DW, Fiore MC, Jorenby DE, et al. Gender differences in smoking cessation. J Consult Clin Psychol 1999;67(4):555-562.

Wileyto EP, Patterson F, Niaura R, et al. Recurrent event analysis of lapse and recovery in a smoking cessation clinical trial using bupropion. Nicotine Tob Res 2005;7(2):257-68.

Zelman DC, Brandon TH, Jorenby DE, et al. Measures of affect and nicotine dependence predict differential response to smoking cessation treatments. J Consult Clin Psychol 1992;60(6):943-952.

Ziedonis D, Harris P, Brandt P, et al. Motivational enhancement therapy and nicotine replacement improve smoking cessation outcomes for smokers with schizophrenia or depression. Addiction 1997:633.

APPENDIX E: ACRONYMS AND ABBREVIATIONS

AE	adverse effects
am	ante meridian (before noon)
BA	behavioral activation
BATS	behavioral activation treatment for smoking
BID	two times per day
BDI-II	Beck Depression Inventory-II
CBT	cognitive behavioral therapy
CES-D	Center for Epidemiologic Studies-Depression
CI	confidence interval
CO	carbon monoxide
DIS	Diagnostic Interview Schedule
FTQ	Fagerstrom Tolerance Questionnaire
FTND	Fagerstrom Test for Nicotine Dependence
GEE	generalized estimating equation
ID	identification
HDRS	Hamilton Depression Rating Scale
ITT	intention to treat
MDD	major depressive disorder
MDE	major depressive episode
mg	milligram or milligrams
mo	month or months
ml	milliliter or milliliters
N or n	number
NA	not applicable
NCI	National Cancer Institute
ng	nanogram
NRT	nicotine replacement therapy
NR	not reported
ns or NS	not significant
OR	odds ratio
p	probability
pm	post meridian (after noon)
POMS	Profile of Mood States
ppm	parts per million
RCT	randomized controlled trial
SCID	Structured Clinical Interview for DSM Diagnoses
SD	standard deviation
SE	standard error
ST	standard treatment
UDD	unipolar depressive disorder
vs	versus
wk	week or weeks
yr	year or years